STRETCHING
&
PREGNANCY

Kit Laughlin with Jennifer Cristaudo

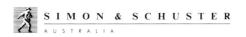

SIMON & SCHUSTER
AUSTRALIA

NOTE TO READERS

This book contains the opinions and ideas of its author. It is intended to provide helpful and informative material on the subjects addressed in the book. It is sold with the understanding that the author and publisher are not engaged in rendering medical, health or any other kind of personal professional services in this book. The reader should consult their medical, health or other competent professional before adopting any of the suggestions in this book or drawing inferences from it.

The author and publisher disclaim all responsibility for any liability, loss or risk, personal or otherwise, which is incurred as a consequence, directly or indirectly, of the use and application of any of the contents of this book.

STRETCHING & PREGNANCY

First published in Australia in 2001
by Simon & Schuster (Australia) Pty Limited
20 Barcoo Street, East Roseville NSW 2069

A Viacom Company
Sydney New York London Toronto Singapore

Text and photographs © Kit Laughlin 2001

National Library of Australia
Cataloguing in Publication data

Laughlin, Kit, 1953- .
Stretching & pregnancy.

Includes index.
ISBN 0 7318 1095 3.

1. Exercise for pregnant women. 2. Mothers - Health and hygiene. 3. Stretching exercises. I. Cristaudo, Jennifer. II. Title.

618.24

Designed by Jeremy Mears
Typeset in 11/13 Garamond
Printed in Singapore by Kyodo Printing Company
10 9 8 7 6 5 4 3 2 1

CONTENTS

Preface

What this book is about

Although *Posture & Flexibility* (*P&F*) is useful for people of all ages and backgrounds, Jennifer Cristaudo and I have long felt there is a definite need for a book that presents certain important aspects of *P&F* specifically for expectant women and for those who have just given birth.

Jennifer is a senior teacher of *P&F*, and in our discussions on various aspects of our work, we have agreed that the two most pressing needs were information on:

- a simple set of *stretching exercises* for those preparing to give birth, and to help the postpartum mother regain her full function; and
- some *relaxation exercises*—to assist both in that seemingly interminable last few weeks before giving giving birth, and in the stressful postpartum period.

In addition to this material on *stretching* and on *relaxation*, we felt that it would be helpful for such a book to include some *birth positions* found useful by Jennifer and the people she has been working with.

Finally, we decided that a *sensible eating plan* was needed—to help postpartum women to get their figures back while feeding two people at the same time.

How this book is set out

The *Introduction* talks about how we have come to the approach that we take in the stretching classes we run—known as *Posture & Flexibility* (*P&F*). The Introduction describes how *P&F* came about, how Jennifer and I met, and the long relationship that has ensued, during which Jennifer has been a senior teacher of *P&F* for many years.

Then I hand over to Jennifer for her to describe her experiences with *P&F* and, in particular, the experiences she had in her own pregnancies and labours. She describes how being flexible and supple helped her during pregnancy and helped her to find a comfortable birth position. In the process of being a senior teacher, Jennifer has worked with many pregnant women herself, and her insights will be useful to you.

Chapter 1 then describes the *prenatal exercises*. These are divided into two parts:
- the *strengthening movements*, including exercises for the ankles, hips, and legs; and
- the *flexibility* exercises.

The bulk of Chapter 1 is devoted to the flexibility exercises—which include various stretches for people of different levels of flexibility and strength. It also includes stretches for parts of the body that are likely to have an adverse effect on your posture during pregnancy, as well as stretches for those muscles in the hips that, if tight, can lead to sciatica-like conditions. Chapter 1 also includes exercises designed to relieve backache.

Chapter 2 describes the *relaxation positions*. The chapter begins with a short section discussing the importance of relaxation and a relaxation script. You could have a friend record this if you wish, or you can obtain a copy from us. (Contact details can be found on page 148.) The audio cassette features a long version of the script read by Kit, with soothing Pacific Ocean sounds in the background; side B features Jennifer reading a shorter version of the script.

The second part of Chapter 2 shows you the most effective relaxation positions. As anyone who is pregnant will know, lying on your back face up (the standard recommended position for relaxation) can be anything but comfortable as the pregnancy progresses. It can also restrict the flow of blood to the placenta, and hence to the foetus. Jennifer will show you some alternative comfortable positions in which you can do your relaxation practice.

The last part of Chapter 2 shows Jennifer's preferred birth positions—which include all of the standard recommendations and a few innovative ones as well.

Chapter 3 discusses *postnatal exercises*, with an emphasis on tightening both the muscles of the pelvic floor and the muscles of the waist, so that you can regain your function and figure as speedily as possible. This is not just a cosmetic consideration. Much recent research has shown that regaining strength in the abdominal 'corset' (as this complex group of muscles is sometimes named) will provide necessary support for the lower back. Everyone knows that back pain is a common occurrence following birth, but few people are aware that the main reason for the back problems is a combination of tightened hip flexor muscles (the muscles that lift your thigh towards your chest) and tightened lumbar (lower back) muscles, together with weakened and lengthened abdominal muscles. Chapter 3 shows you how to regain the strength in the abdominal muscles and how to stretch the tight muscles very effectively.

Chapter 4, the final chapter in the book, is a discussion of what we have found to be the most effective dietary recommendations—bearing in mind the need for adequate nutrition for the foetus before birth, the desire to breastfeed effectively after delivery, and the importance of regaining your former shape after pregnancy and labour. The path to good nutrition and maximising lean muscle mass (as the jargon has it these days) is a simple, commonsense approach to eating that is both delicious and nutritious.

After the main text has concluded, we have a short section summarising how to use the book (*Putting It All Together*) followed by a selected list of *References and Reading List*. The reference list is by no means exhaustive. There are so many books on the subjects covered in the present book that a full list would take many pages. We have chosen those books that we believe will be practical and useful to you.

Finally, we include *Contact Details* (for those of you who wish to make personal contact with us) and two *Indexes*. There is a short conventional index of major topics discussed, but because a *word index* of exercises has limitations in a book about positions of the body (positions that are hard to express in a few words), a *visual* index of exercises is also presented. This consists of a collection of small photographs showing the end positions of each exercise and including a page number and an exercise number to help you find the exercise that you are seeking. Once you know which of the exercises you would like to practise, this visual index will be the easiest way to find it at a subsequent practice session.

How to use this book

Choose what you need

The Introduction covers the development of the system that has come to be known as *Posture & Flexibility* (*P&F*), and goes on to describe how Jennifer and I met and our ongoing involvement with *P&F*. If this is of no particular interest to you, you can proceed directly to Chapter 1, providing that you first read the sections on 'General cautions' (page 5) and 'Specific cautions' (page 5).

I assume that a variety of people will be using this book, including those planning a family and those who have just recently given birth. You can turn to whichever section of the book that you feel is most appropriate to your particular situation.

However, if you are planning a family some time in the future, the sooner that you do the right stretching exercises the better. If you have just given birth, the strengthening exercises will be of most interest to you.

Read before trying!

We strongly recommend that the text accompanying any particular exercise or any photograph be read completely before attempting the positions shown. There are many safety issues of relevance here. Particular ways of breathing, ways of holding yourself, and specific work to do in each position is contained in the text—rather than in the captions under the photographs. Therefore, for both safety and effectiveness, you should read all of the text before you attempt any exercise.

When to exercise

We recommend that you exercise as far as possible at the same time each day. Experience has shown that you are far more likely to do your exercises if you make a definite decision to exercise at a particular time each day, rather than saying to yourself you will fit it in 'at some time'.

We have found that the body is loosest in the evenings, so this is the time to do stretches that are hardest for you.

Stretching exercise is best done a couple of hours or more after your last main meal, so reserving some time in the evening for your practice is a good idea. Of course, if you are feeling a bit hungry and faint have something light to eat or drink before exercising.

If you are planning your practice routine on a weekly basis, we suggest that the stretching exercises be done a few days each week, and only the relaxation exercises on another couple of days a week. If you find that you have enough time to be able to do the relaxation exercises following the three practice sessions of stretching exercise each week, so much the better. We have found that combining the relaxation with the stretching provides the best possible effects overall, but we are also mindful that many people are very busy and that time is often a constraint. Be realistic about what you can achieve in any given day.

Warmth and clothing

A warm-to-medium-hot bath can make your body move more freely. So if you find that your body is at the stiffer end of the spectrum, use a bath to help warm-up your muscles, ligaments, and associated tissues. A shower will not be as effective.

Wearing reasonably warm clothing will also help. Research in Germany has shown that a rise in the core temperature of a muscle of one to two degrees Celsius increases the flexibility of that joint and its associated muscles by 15–20%—a considerable increase. Wear clothing that is warm and that permits free movement. Tight clothing can inhibit the possible range of movement of your body to a surprising extent.

Avoid interruptions

To avoid unnecessary interruptions, and as a matter of safety and comfort, it is essential to go to the toilet before attempting any stretching exercises. This becomes even more important as your pregnancy advances.

We also suggest that you pull the phone out of the wall or put a pillow over it—to avoid being interrupted for the fifteen or twenty minutes of your practice. This is especially important if you decide to do the relaxation practice as well. Nothing will be as disturbing as the sound of a phone while you are trying to relax!

Similarly, keep house pets away—it is just not possible to stretch while your dog is climbing all over you! This recommendation goes for young children as well, unless they are old enough to join you in your practice.

We feel that it is essential for an expectant woman to have a little bit of time by herself each day, and your stretching and relaxation practice might as well be that time. In other words, be nice to yourself and make a little bit of time just for you.

Aids and props

While exercising, make sure that you have a tea towel and a strap or belt (or something similar) handy. We will use props of this nature—as well as cushions, blankets and so on—to make the final position a little easier to achieve.

Again, it is a good idea to read through any given exercise before you attempt it. You will then be aware of the props that you might need to do the exercise most effectively.

The importance of 'form'

When you are trying a stretching exercise yourself, please imitate the *form* of the exercise as Jennifer is practising it—rather than her *performance* of any particular exercise. For example, rather than just trying to take your head towards your knees in a forwards-bending exercise, try to understand exactly what the exercise is *trying* to achieve, the muscles that the exercise is meant to stretch, and what work you must do to ensure *good form*. If you do manage to imitate the *form* of an exercise properly, the benefits are hugely improved.

Listen to your body

The most important suggestion is probably the most subtle. It is to *listen* to what your body is telling you as you do this work, especially if you are new to stretching exercises. There is a wealth of understanding to be gained from your own body, but it is an understanding to which most of us in our Western culture are least sensitive. This cannot be learnt from a book or from a video—it is unique to every individual, and no teacher can see what is going on inside your body.

Even if Jennifer and I were practising the exercises with you, we would still be urging you to have most of your attention focused *inside* your body to receive this important information. Attending to this sensory flow will enhance the experience of any kind of exercise, and also makes the doing of the exercise much safer.

If you are new to doing stretching exercise, you don't want to be too sore the next day, so it is better to do too little rather than too much. You can always make the next session a little more intense.

Listen to your body, and adjust the content and the length of your exercise session accordingly.

General cautions

Please ensure that you discuss any medical conditions or any other concerns with your medical practitioner. If you feel any unusual discomfort, discontinue your practice, and recommence only after you have received the 'all-clear' from your doctor or midwife.

Do the exercises that you feel comfortable with, and approach each exercise using commonsense. Adjust your practice depending on the way that you feel. Sometimes there are exercises that you will not feel comfortable doing—for example, if you are feeling nauseous, tired, or dizzy.

Lying on your back can feel quite uncomfortable, especially in the later stages of pregnancy as your baby becomes bigger. It can also be dangerous for you and your baby. In this position, the weight of the baby can restrict blood flow to the placenta and to your own brain. It is therefore not recommended that you spend much time in this position. If you feel light-headed or dizzy, you should certainly stop doing exercises in this position.

Specific cautions

Placenta praevia

If you have placenta praevia, avoid strenuous exercise, although gentle stretching is fine.

You will find specific *contractions* described in many of the exercises below. However, if you have placenta praevia you should *not* perform these parts of the described exercises.

Avoid full squats. If you really want to practise this pose, ensure that you sit on a support such as a low stool or similar.

Varicosities

Varicosities can occur in any part of your body. They are a result of relaxin (a hormone that softens connective tissue during pregnancy), the physical stress of supporting extra weight and, possibly, poor circulation.

If you have varicosities, it is important to rest and try to improve your circulation by exercising gently. Take weight off your feet and elevate your legs where possible.

If anal and vaginal varicosities are a problem, concentrate on pelvic-floor exercises to tone these muscles and improve circulation (see the beginning of Chapter 3, page 101). Avoid full squats and ensure that you use a stool if you wish to continue this exercise.

Vaginal prolapse

The advice for vaginal prolapse is similar to that for varicosities, although your practitioner might recommend that you avoid squats and strong legs-apart stretches altogether.

If prolapse is a problem, you must focus on pelvic-floor exercises, so practise these religiously.

Blood pressure

Blood pressure problems can be due to high or low blood pressure.

If your blood pressure is *high*, avoid exercises that place your head lower than your heart. Try to breathe evenly, and relax in all stretches. Leave out any stretches that you feel affect you adversely. Concentrate especially on your relaxation and breathing. Don't overdo things.

Low blood pressure can mean that you feel faint if you stand for long periods, or if you stand up quickly. Avoid stretches that place your head lower than your heart, and try to come out of each stretch slowly, breathing in as you come up. You might need to move from the floor to a standing position, so practise next to sturdy furniture that gives you something to hold on to. If you do feel particularly dizzy, lie down, breathe, relax, and get up when you feel better. Don't forget to eat!

Separated abdominal muscles

If your medical practitioner has diagnosed that your abdominal muscles (the *rectus abdominis* muscles) have separated, you can do gentle strengthening exercises while you are pregnant (with professional approval). If you feel uncomfortable doing these or have any concerns about doing these while pregnant, concentrate on correcting this condition postpartum. The exercises are found in Chapter 3.

Although this a not a dangerous condition, it is best to avoid stretches that put undue stress on these muscles. Avoid or reduce rotations, sideways bending, and backwards bending.

Amniocentesis

Amniocentesis is a physically invasive diagnostic test. It is advisable to discontinue stretching for a short period after this test and recommence your practice after consultation with your doctor.

Breech presentation

If your baby is confirmed as a breech presentation (that is, a position with the baby's head uppermost and the tail lower), avoid squatting. You can recommence if the baby turns and engages normally.

Cervical stitch (Shirodkar suture)

If you have a cervical stitch (otherwise known as a Shirodkar suture) inserted, avoid full squatting. Discuss other stretches with your medical practitioner. Avoid using contractions in the exercises.

Lower-back and/or intervertebral disc problems

If you have lower-back and/or intervertebral disc problems, discuss intended exercises with your medical practitioner. Most will recommend gentle stretching.

As your posture changes during pregnancy, there is a tendency for the curve of the lower back to become more accentuated. A number of the chair exercises can relieve the discomfort of this change (Exercises 5, 6, and 7), and the hip-flexor and quadriceps exercises (Exercises 11, 14, and 15) can reduce the tendency to an exaggerated lumbar curve.

For more detailed suggestions, consult our companion volume *Overcome Neck & Back Pain.*

IVF pregnancies or threat of miscarriage

If you have an IVF pregnancy, or are suffering from a threatened miscarriage, discontinue stretches. Recommence after consultation with your medical practitioner. Do not use contractions in the exercises.

INTRODUCTION

Pregnancy and *P&F*

The *Posture & Flexibility* (*P&F*) classes have now been running at the Australian National University (ANU) for thirteen years and, in that time, we have had a huge variety of students. Past and present class members include teenagers who have just begun their first year in university, the professionals who work at the university (including lecturers, technicians, and researchers), and the 'Over 40s' class.

The classes contain almost equal numbers of men and women. From time to time, students have advised me that they are pregnant and have wondered whether doing the exercises that we routinely do in the classes are safe during pregnancy. I have reassured them, but I have added that, although we always suggest that *all* students do their exercises carefully, someone who is expecting a child needs to take even more care.

Over the years we have had many requests for modifications of our standard exercises—especially as pregnancy advances and certain positions become uncomfortable or simply impossible due to the size of the abdomen. Our national *P&F* organiser, Mrs Sharon Clark (herself a mother of two), has had many enquiries by telephone and through our website as to whether our exercises are safe for expectant women. And we have had a number of enquiries from various bodywork practitioners—including teachers of yoga, Pilates, Alexander Technique, Feldencrais, massage practitioners, chiropractors, and osteopaths.

The common thread to all the enquiries—from women expecting a child or from practitioners who work with them—was the perceived need for a book that dealt with stretching exercises in a non-technical way, and that had adaptations of various standard stretching positions that were especially suitable for pregnant women. Because of the desire for a non-technical approach, the present book contains no detailed descriptions or illustrations of the anatomy involved in particular stretches, apart from information that is absolutely necessary for safe or effective execution of any particular stretch. Readers looking for more detailed information on exercises suitable for neck or back problems will find the book *Overcome Neck & Back Pain* helpful. Those who wish to have more detailed anatomical and technical information in relation to the widest possible range of stretches will find this in the companion publication *Stretching & Flexibility*.

There is a companion videotape to this book (also entitled *Stretching & Pregnancy*) in which Jennifer demonstrates all of the recommended exercises. You might find that watching the video, and imitating her movements, is an easier way to learn.

A further source of useful information is our website <www.posture-and-flexibility.com.au>.

How *P&F* began

The genesis for *Posture & Flexibility* was my four-year stay in Japan where, as a thirty-year-old television director, I found myself in an unfamiliar, complex culture. It was much like being a child again. I found myself unable to speak the language, unable to read simple bus or shop signs, and surrounded by a very large group of people who looked quite different from me. Everything had to be learnt anew, and I needed to rely on people's assistance in ways large and small. My foreignness was something of which I was aware every day, and was a salutary lesson in cultural sensitivity for someone who comes from a European background living in Australia.

The most important aspect of this experience of feeling child-like in Japan was the absolute necessity of questioning the most fundamental assumptions I had about how the world works. I had to reassess my values anew. I had to ask myself which values were important to me, and which were not. In short, my entire world view was challenged. The benefit of this experience for an adult cannot be overestimated, and the extensive amount of work I did on my way of thinking, and my physical self, came to be reflected in the *P&F* approach to doing body work.

Some features of *P&F*

Essential criteria

The two essential criteria for assessing *P&F* routines are that they must be *effective* and they must be *safe*.

In starting from scratch in devising a system for helping adults to become more flexible, I needed to be certain that the recommendations that I was making for my students were *effective*—that is, that they would provide tangible changes for the individuals using them.

Apart from effectiveness, the other criterion, as noted above, was the absolute necessity for *safety*. Over the thirteen years that *P&F* has been operating at the ANU, we have abandoned almost as many forms as we now teach, which number approximately one hundred exercises.

This process of selecting and refining has facilitated the development of a robust body of work. *P&F* differs from a number of schools of body work in important ways.

How *P&F* differs

Turning inwards

First among these differences is our insistence, from the very first lesson, that students turn their attention *inwards* to what is actually going in inside their own bodies. In this way, students commence a 'dialogue' with their internal selves. This dialogue matures over time and gives our students insights into their internal affairs that cannot be gained in any other way.

Turning students' direction inwards in this way also makes the doing of the exercises considerably safer than it would be if their attention were focused on some external goal—such as becoming more flexible. In my view, the acquisition of this internal understanding is of much greater value than any demonstrable external flexibility.

Without question, this approach is also the best way to overcome any pain or discomfort in your body.

An anatomical basis

Another important aspect of our work is the insistence that there be an anatomical reason for doing stretches in a particular way.

P&F is thus scientifically based. This anatomical basis for all *P&F* exercises means that everything we do has a sound rationale for what we are attempting to achieve and how we are attempting to achieve it.

Key practical elements of *P&F*

Let us now look at the key elements of *P&F* in actually doing the exercises.

The key elements that distinguish the *P&F* approach from other approaches to stretching are as follows.
- We pay particular attention to what we call 'form'.
- We use the *Contract–Relax* (*C–R*) approach.
- We use this *C–R* approach within a structure of *partial poses.*
- Some of these *partial poses* are *partner-assisted.*

Some thoughts on each of these are offered below.

Form

The archetypal stretch exercise in *P&F* holds your body in a particular position and moves it in a certain way to stretch a nominated muscle group. Approaching a stretch in this way draws attention to what we call 'form'—in other words, the way that the body must be held or moved to isolate a particular muscle group.

Students are asked to move gently into a position until they can feel a stretching sensation in the target muscle group. This is the first step and is common to all exercises. The starting position typically is held for five to thirty seconds—until the person feels comfortable in this new position. For many people, just getting into a stretch position will always feel a little strange at first!

Contract–Relax (*C–R*)

The second element of our approach in actually doing the exercises is to use the *Contract–Relax* (*C–R*) technique.

From any stretch position, a gentle isometric ('same length') contraction is performed. This requires the student to push or pull the muscle being stretched. No movement of the limb being used to provide this force is allowed. This contraction is typically held for three to thirty seconds—the length of time depending on the size of the muscle group being worked. We have found that the larger the muscle group, the longer the contraction necessary to provide an adequate second stretch.

In some exercises, this resistance for the isometric contraction is provided by a partner's weight, or strength, or body part.

The student then stops the contraction, takes in a breath and, *while breathing out*, performs a second stretch (what we call a 're-stretch').

Those of you who have not tried this *C–R* approach will not appreciate the extent to which a small gentle isometric contraction completely changes the sensation of going into the second stretch position. The new stretch position—typically 5–15 degrees further in the range of movement being practised—is then held for a number of breaths, letting the body relax as much as possible. Typically, the suggested number of breaths ranges from three to ten. Here again, the larger the muscle group the longer the recommended second stretch position.

To summarise, once the student is in a stretch position, a contraction is performed. This activates the muscles being stretched. The contraction is stopped, a breath is taken in, and the whole body relaxed (except for those parts required to hold the form or the position). Then a second stretch is done.

Among the many advantages of using the *C–R* approach is that muscles that are typically very difficult to identify in your own body (such as the hip flexors), will make their presence known to you instantly. Another advantage is that the contraction provides an immediate alteration in the way your brain maps the tension in the muscle being stretched, and the sensation of tightness in a particular muscle group can be altered by just one or two contractions in a single stretch session.

Another advantage of the *C–R* approach is that, unlike other approaches to stretching, your strength at the end of the range of movement improves. This is due to the isometric strengthening effect—which has been the subject of much research over the last twenty or thirty years.

We have tested most of the current methods available to the Western world with regard to improving flexibility, and can confidently say that the *C–R* approach is the safest and most efficient.

Partial poses

The *partial poses* aspect of our approach is absolutely essential for beginning students.

In a typical (non-*P&F*) exercise class, it is common for a teacher to require students to try to fold their bodies forwards over their legs while sitting with their legs stretched out in front of them. As many of you will know, this is an extremely difficult movement to do in good form—'good form' being the requirement to hold the spine in a neutral or straight shape. In fact, this particular exercise requires extreme flexibility in the hamstrings and is really an advanced exercise.

In *P&F*, we introduce a *partial pose* to assist beginners. An example of a partial pose is to fold one of your legs (thus taking one leg out of the stretching equation) and to use the strength of your trunk to hold your back straight. This means that the hamstrings of *only one* of your legs are stretched at a time. This reduces the discomfort of the stretch and allows you to compare one side with the other.

A further innovation is that, using the present example exercise, it is possible to get an extremely effective stretch in your hamstring muscles while having the knee of the leg that you are stretching slightly bent. This almost completely reduces the 'alarm sensation' from the muscle being stretched, and allows you to relax into the position. Further, doing contractions with the hamstrings of the bent leg and then using the quadriceps (the muscles at the front of your thigh) to straighten the leg further, we are using a number of well-researched reflexes to aid improvements in flexibility. *Doing a stretching exercise in which a joint can be moved from bent to straight is the most effective way to improve your flexibility.*

Another example of our use of partial poses is the use of a hip (*piriformis*) stretch or a calf muscle stretch before trying to stretch your hamstrings. A beginning student will not realise the extent to which tightness in these two muscle groups can profoundly influence the capacity to bend forwards at the hips with a straight back and straight legs.

All of these aspects will be covered in the exercise themselves. They are all examples of what we mean when we use the term 'partial pose'.

Partners

In our *P&F* stretching classes, we use *partners* a great deal. In the present book, Jennifer and I decided to show the exercises as solo stretches. We did this because many expectant women might not be able to work out with somebody else. However, if you *do* have someone to practise with, you can find a stronger version (a 'partner version') of all of the exercises in the companion volume *Stretching & Flexibility*.

We recommend practising with someone else if you can. Not only is this more enjoyable, but also it allows a much stricter attention to form (see page 11). Your partner becomes your second pair of eyes, and can give you the feedback that your body might not be able to give—especially for those who are less experienced with these exercises.

Some final thoughts on *P&F*

P&F has challenged assumptions. For example, the assumption that there is a need for daily stretching has been challenged because we have found that stretching every day is simply not necessary if you wish to become flexible—especially as an adult. Two or three short stretching sessions a week are all that anyone needs to become more flexible. I imagine that this will be very welcome news to expectant women, for whom 'spare time' is more of an amusing concept than a reality!

Overall, we see effective stretching as a kind of self-maintenance that can be done anywhere and at any time. I envisage an era when stretching, and the teaching of stretching, will be unnecessary, because individuals will have this kind of understanding about how their bodies work. As a culture, we have an extraordinary depth of understanding into natural processes *outside* ourselves. We understand chemistry, biology, physics, and all sorts of other academic and practical enquiry. But it seems clear to me—from years of clinical and academic experience, and from the experience of teaching stretching exercises to many thousands of people—that the least-valued area of knowledge is that understanding that can be gained only by working on ourselves. *P&F* is a partial attempt to solve the problem of how we might understand ourselves better, and how we might understand how we fit into something larger than ourselves.

Some readers have commented that the exercises we recommend look like yoga poses, or exercises from traditional martial arts, or gymnastics, or dance. The fact is that there are only so many ways in which the body can be moved and positioned, and many schools of body work have converged on the same solutions. Of all the schools of body work extant, I believe that some schools of yoga are the most complete—but all of them lack specific exercises for particular muscle groups. We have tried to design stretches that allow individuals (sometimes assisted by a partner) to explore, safely and effectively, the stretching sensation in all muscle groups in their bodies.

Introducing Jennifer

We shot the last of the prenatal exercises on the Friday (and they happened to be the most difficult ones). Jennifer was looking very pregnant—about eight months and a week (or possibly two, she thought). So I was not especially surprised when she didn't turn up to the following Tuesday's Advanced Class—the one that all teachers attend.

When I rang her house, her partner, Chris, answered.

'Jennifer wasn't at class last night, and she didn't have a note from her mother!' I joked.

'She was in hospital, giving birth to Pernille!' replied Chris.

'That's just not good enough!'

We both laughed.

'How long was her labour?' I asked.

'Two hours.'

'She has a casual attitude about everything she does,' I observed.

We both laughed again.

This little story encapsulates some of the many qualities of Jennifer, one of the two senior *P&F* teachers at the ANU.

I met Jennifer about twelve years ago when she was one of the first students in my early classes run at the Sports Union at the ANU. Jennifer had many impressive characteristics, of which her temperament was the most outstanding. She was (and is) unfailingly pleasant and genuinely caring for the people around her. In addition to these personal characteristics, Jennifer had an aptitude for stretching and made very rapid progress indeed. In only about a year she was assisting me in the classes and I asked her to consider teaching a Beginners' class.

Jennifer has been teaching *P&F* at the ANU and other locations for nine or ten years now and she has been one of our two senior instructors for the past five years. This reflects her considerable organisational talent, and her contributions to *P&F*.

Jennifer's greatest contribution to the enterprise, however, is in her capacity to teach people how to teach. In addition to her tertiary qualifications in this area she has a natural talent. She embodies all the teaching virtues—being kind, genuinely interested in her students, having good listening skills, and being always available to talk.

When I originally had the idea for making a video of exercises for expectant women, it was natural to turn to Jennifer for assistance (apart from the fact that she was about six or seven months pregnant at the time!). We have had many discussions about the contents of this book. Although my experience in this area is limited, it is true to say that the general principles of *P&F* can be applied to any task where flexibility is desirable. Once we had started shooting the video it seemed quite natural to shoot the stills for a book at the same time. From there, it was a small step to begin to write the text for this book—although a much larger one to finish!

In the following section Jennifer will talk about her own experiences with *P&F*, and the experiences of giving birth with such short labours—two and a half hours for Anreas and two hours for Pernille. Of course, we are not claiming that being flexible was the sole reason for these easy deliveries—but it certainly helped.

Jennifer writes

Advantages of being flexible

What are the advantages of being flexible? Quite simply, flexibility is imperative to keep your body functioning at its optimum level. Stretching releases physical tension, and having muscles that are soft and relaxed means that your body remains supple. Being flexible also reduces the risk of injury and aids in the recuperation of existing injury. As a result, you can enjoy a sense of *empowerment*—knowing that you can actually control and significantly contribute to your own physical wellbeing.

When you stretch and become more flexible you come to know your body and its capabilities. With this knowledge you can address your individual strengths and weaknesses. Your body is a remarkable piece of machinery and can be readily trained. If you begin stretching, and continue to stretch, there is no doubt that you will become more flexible.

Many people do not really 'live in' their bodies—unlike children who delight in the wondrous things that their bodies allow them to do. Years of conditioning, both social and physical, can cause you to be at at odds with your shape, your size, your weight, the way you look, and the way that you feel about yourself. Rediscovering your body and feeling all the muscles you never knew you had, will be a remarkable journey for you—just as your pregnancy will be.

As your baby continues to grow and your body changes, doing these exercises will help to 'centre' you and keep you focused on this incredible transformation. Stretching will also help you to get to know your body, and the most important benefit of this is the realisation that your body has a remarkable ability to heal itself.

As you learn to stretch you begin to understand that you can work through discomfort or pain. If you do have a strained muscle you realise that it will heal with time. Most importantly, however, you learn to *trust* your body, and this is the most beneficial outcome of all. As you approach labour it is important to be confident and know that you have physically prepared yourself to the best of your ability. When the momentous occasion of giving birth comes, you will have the tools to help you relax, to move freely, and to 'breathe' your baby into the world.

Beware of overstretching

At this point, however, it is important to caution you against *overstretching*. During pregnancy the hormone relaxin is at work to help soften muscles and ligaments throughout the body. As a result, joints also become more mobile and you gain flexibility faster during pregnancy than you otherwise would. Although the expansion of the pelvis is a natural and necessary part of pregnancy, overstretching of the hips and pelvis is to be avoided. If you find, as I did in my first pregnancy, that your sacroiliac joints (where the spine joins the pelvis) are too mobile, I suggest that you continue to do the hip stretches gently, monitor your progress, and adjust your zeal accordingly.

As an aside, most of my students and I often find that we do not feel the full effects of a stretching session on the day after. Rather, we become aware of it on the day after that.

Please take note of your reactions to stretches. It might be helpful to keep a diary. Write down the exercises that you do and any other notes you wish to make, including your physical and emotional responses to each stretch.

The teacher learns!

I have been teaching *P&F* since late 1992—the same year that I completed my postgraduate Diploma of Teaching. Teaching in high schools and colleges, and teaching the *P&F* classes at the ANU, have led me to the conclusion that my best teachers have been my own students. As a teacher, I find I am constantly challenged by my students and it is they who demand that I exceed my own expectations and abilities. It would be fair to say, however, that I am more successful on some days than on others!

Working with pregnant students is especially rewarding. Because the vast majority are already students of *P&F*, they have a 'head start' as they are familiar with many of the stretches. These students also seem to adapt readily to their physical changes and know their limits in terms of flexibility. However, it is not essential to have this prior knowledge. Anyone who is diligent and mindful of their movements and activities will be equally rewarded.

Exercises for pregnant women

At the ANU we do not offer classes especially designed for pregnant women. The main reason for this is that in all of our classes there is a constant need to modify stretches to suit each individual. In this respect, the needs of pregnant women are not so different from the various needs of other individual students.

Some of my pregnant students have been very flexible, but not strong. Others have had injuries (unrelated to their pregnancies) that must be dealt with accordingly. Others have had pregnancy-related health conditions that have an impact on the kinds of exercises they can perform. In short, all of these needs are as individual as the women themselves, pregnant or otherwise.

It is important to view pregnancy as a normal physical state. There is no real need to have pregnant women segregated into their own classes. They are as able-bodied as any other student. They are just pregnant!

Consequently, all of the exercises in this book are standard *P&F* exercises that are taught in all of our classes. Although the exercises are 'standard' *P&F* exercises, many of the exercises in this book are variations of existing stretches, and some of these modifications have been specifically designed for our pregnant students. The process of modifying exercises is fairly straightforward and simply involves the student and teacher playing around with different ideas until we come up with something to suit the individual.

This challenge continues as the needs of each woman change during the course of her pregnancy. What she feels comfortable doing in the early stages of pregnancy, and what she is actually capable of doing towards the end of pregnancy, can be quite different!

The relationship between student and teacher is therefore egalitarian, and involves trust and mutual respect by both parties. In this regard, all of my students, and not just the pregnant ones, are to be applauded for trusting me as their teacher and allowing me to lead them into sometimes uncharted waters.

Exercises for labour

Being strong and flexible is also important if you want to be active while in labour. Most of my students plan to give birth at home or in birthing centres where freedom of movement is encouraged.

As a general rule, we focus on loosening the muscles in and around your hips to help 'open' the pelvis. Most students who want to deliver in a squat or semi-squat position work hard at building up their leg strength. They also concentrate on improving their calf and ankle flexibility in particular. You might find that there are other muscle groups you want to focus on.

Knowing how to relax and breathe is important during labour. When you are in pain your first reaction is to recoil and tense up. For example, if you jam your finger in a door, you quickly pull back, hold the hand close to your body, and double over. Learning to relax in the face of pain—indeed, learning to 'embrace' the pain—will help you enormously when you deliver your baby.

I have been lucky enough in my life never to have experienced severe pain apart from childbirth. I have never broken a bone, been in a serious accident, or undergone surgery. It is therefore difficult for me to discuss the pain of labour with reference to any other pain experience. I suspect that this is a pointless exercise anyway.

When approaching labour, even if this is not your first baby, it is important to remember that each delivery is different. It is also important to accept that your labour, in real terms, will be beyond your control. Your acceptance of this, along with the knowledge that you have done your best to prepare for this experience, is imperative.

Being healthy, strong, fit, and flexible is the best way to prepare yourself physically. Being calm, confident, and emotionally open is possibly even more important. Practising these exercises will help you to focus, to relax, and to breathe—the basic steps towards an empowered labour.

Postpartum exercises

Postpartum flexibility means that you can enjoy, with minimal physical stress, the hard physical labour that goes with parenting. As you become used to performing exercises on the floor—finding yourself in odd positions and being comfortable moving freely— you will really reap the benefits. Children spend most of their time on the floor playing and rolling around, and being more flexible means that you can join in their fun.

Think about the kinds of movements that are related to parenting. How many times a day does the average parent need to bend down, pick up, reach over, lift, carry, and set down again? If you do not have the required strength and flexibility your body will rebel. No matter how strong you are, carrying a baby on one arm, and doing everything else with the other, can be very tiring (not to mention challenging!). Knowing how to stretch those tight, sore muscles yourself not only will help you on a day-to-day level, but also will save you having to pay someone else to do it for you.

Being flexible is imperative in avoiding aches, pains, strains, and injuries. If you have undergone a Caesarean section, ensure that you stretch carefully only after consultation with your surgeon.

Doing the exercises

How far into pregnancy?

The prenatal sections of both this book and the associated video were shot in the last trimester of my second pregnancy, between weeks 35 and 37. We finished shooting on a Friday and I delivered Peri (eighteen days early) on the following Tuesday. In both pregnancies I continued to stretch and teach right up to the delivery dates. In fact, I felt so well that in both pregnancies I almost attended the Advanced class to have a stretch myself on the nights that I gave birth (but I went into labour instead!).

Stasis is the enemy of a supple body. Movement, in any form, is paramount in keeping joints and muscles loose. If you are tired and feel uncomfortable and cumbersome, especially in the later stages of your pregnancy, simply do what you can and rest as often as you need. Remember that every aspect of your pregnancy is just a stage which, in reality, will pass all too quickly. Take time to reflect on the marvellous changes that are happening to you. Relax and enjoy!

Advantages of stretching

Apart from the various advantages already mentioned, stretching might also help to alleviate some of the more common physical stresses of pregnancy by loosening muscles and making you more aware of your posture. This voyage of physical self-discovery will help you to learn to trust your body and know what you are capable of doing. This 'body confidence' will be invaluable as you prepare for labour.

Stretching also allows you to have some emotional 'time out' to listen to your body. This is particularly important in pregnancy as you need time to adapt to the changes you are experiencing—both physically and emotionally.

Clothing and location

Choose something comfortable to wear. Your clothing should allow free movement but not be too voluminous—you don't want to get tangled up! If you wear a bra, ensure you are properly fitted for a maternity bra so your breasts have good support.

We all dream of having a room of our own for exercising, but often this is not physically possible. You do need a bit of floor space and access to some props—but that's all.

When to exercise

Stretching should be integrated into your lifestyle, and not be seen as a separate activity you do at a special time under perfect conditions. Perfect conditions simply do not exist in most busy households! Certainly make time to have a serious stretch on a regular basis, but all of these exercises can be done almost anywhere and at any time—while watching television, on the floor reading a newspaper, or playing with the kids. Anything is better than nothing, especially in the early days of stretching before a domestic routine is established.

The time of day at which you choose to stretch is dependent on your routine. Some people bounce out of bed in the mornings with bundles of energy. If this sounds like you, mornings might suit you best. Afternoons or evenings are also a good time because they offer a chance to wind down at the end of the day when the body is looser after the day's activities. Stretching after a bath is ideal because your body is generally warmer, and you therefore have a 'head start'.

These exercises can be relaxing but some are quite strenuous. Some help to build strength and improve balance and coordination. Although stretching can be quite invigorating you might end up feeling a little weary, so don't stretch when you are overtired—you might find it hard to concentrate on what you are doing and you don't want to injure yourself. If you are tired and want to unwind before bedtime, try some of the more gentle and relaxing stretches. They will calm you mentally and physically, and you might find that you sleep better as a result. Alternatively, you might omit the stretching exercises, and do only the relaxation exercise from Chapter 2. If you are using the audiotape, there is a short one (about 15 minutes) and a longer one (about 25 minutes).

Monitoring your progress

With all of these exercises it is important to 'listen' to your body and concentrate on how your muscles feel. Move into each stretch gently and slowly and stop before you begin to feel a strong stretch sensation. This will give your muscles time to warm-up so you can relax into the stretch. It will also mean that you do not overstretch. When you feel you can stretch further, do so.

When you first start your practice, try to stay in the stretch for about eight to ten reasonable, ordinary breaths. If you find that you cannot stay in a stretch for very long, it probably means that you are overstretching. Muscles need time to warm-up, and if you are not in a stretched position for a sufficient period of time you are defeating the purpose! Later, as you become more experienced and are more aware of how your body responds to these stretches, you can stretch for longer if you feel comfortable in doing so. You can always do an exercise and then come back and repeat it when you are looser, and able to stay in that position for longer.

I suggest that you monitor your progress carefully and do the stretches that suit you and your level of flexibility. If you have significant pain, or if you are concerned at all, you should speak with your medical practitioner. Some women also find that osteopathy relieves such conditions very effectively.

Some personal reflections

My pregnancies

Both my pregnancies were healthy and normal and I experienced no morning sickness—just a low level of queasiness in the first trimester of each. I felt more tired the first time around, and put this down to teaching fulltime at college, as well as two *P&F* classes each week at the ANU.

I walked to school each day (about forty minutes five times a week) and continued to walk our dog as well. This was my only form of exercise at the time, but it helped to keep me fit and also alleviated a lot of the sacral pain (at the bottom of the spine) that I started to experience at the end of the second trimester.

During my first pregnancy, I did not alter my stretching routine at all and continued to do all the usual stretches—including many more challenging ones that are not in this book. In retrospect, I believe that my sacral discomfort (which at times was quite extreme) was caused by hypermobility in my sacroiliac joints.

In my first pregnancy I was also advised to stop any squatting movements. The midwives were unsure of the position of the baby and believed that he might have been breech. They feared that squatting might encourage the baby to engage in this position, and I could recommence squatting only after they had established that he was not breech.

In my second pregnancy, I did very few hip and groin stretches or strong 'legs-apart' poses as part of my regular stretching sessions. I also avoided lying on my back because I found that doing so, even with my knees pointing up to the ceiling, was too stressful on the sacrum. After excluding these positions, I experienced no sacral pain whatsoever.

My labours

Both my labours were fairly quick. With my first pregnancy, I experienced some mild labour pains in the middle of the night eight days before he was due. The pains did not last long and I promptly went back to sleep. After discussion with my midwife on the following day I decided that it was simply a practice run or 'phantom labour'. I had convinced myself, for some unknown reason, that I would be overdue.

On the following night I felt the 'phantom pains' again. They became stronger and stronger and I went to lie down after about an hour. In retrospect all the signs were there but, as a clueless 'first-timer', it never occurred to me that this was it! Everything after that was just a blur!

My waters broke and it seemed I immediately went into the second stage of labour. I instinctively found myself on all fours with my hips up and my shoulders down in an effort to slow my labour down. However, the labour progressed very rapidly. We hadn't packed anything in preparation for the birth, but my partner Chris coped extremely well. He ran from one room to another, and back to me again, patting me on the back and offering encouragement.

'You're doing really well,' he said. 'Great job.'

The only strict instruction I gave him was to pack a rock melon! He wisely declined to argue, and packed it as asked!

We got to the birth centre with twenty minutes to spare and Anreas was delivered with me in a kneeling position as I leant against the bed, although I had a break at some point and stood in a supported squat. In total, the labour had taken about three hours.

The lead-up to my daughter's birth was quite different although the labour itself was very similar—short and intense. This time my waters broke at 1.30 a.m. eighteen days before the due date. It was 'all systems go' as we hurried down to the birth centre. But nothing happened! My labour failed to establish.

Back home again, we waited for something, anything, to happen. It was the longest day of our lives! We went down to the birth centre at 3 p.m. for a follow-up appointment. Still nothing happened. Home again. Nothing. By this stage I was tired and frustrated.

My contractions eventually started at 9.30 that evening and established quite rapidly. Peri was born at 11.41 that evening and I delivered her in a kneeling position, leaning into an enormous but firm bean bag. I found my relaxation techniques particularly helpful during this labour. I became aware that I was tensing up with each contraction. Making a conscious effort to relax, especially through the stomach muscles, helped me to avoid any unnecessary tension.

In terms of pain relief, some women say that they do not like the effects of gas (nitrous oxide). One friend of mine found it disorientating and described the feeling as being ' . . . outside my head . . . I like being in my head and not separate from my body!'

In this respect, I found that concentrating on my breathing helped me to focus on the intense sensations that I was experiencing. If you want to be 'in your body' during labour, concentrating on your breathing will certainly help to 'centre' you.

I believe that the speed of both my labours was due largely to my level of flexibility, my regular practice, and my basic level of strength. General good health and a positive attitude should not be discounted either.

I can't guarantee that practising these exercises, no matter how diligently, will ensure you a quick labour. But I do believe that you will be empowered through your practice and will come to a better understanding of your body—and these things cannot fail to help.

Resting during pregnancy

Because I was working fulltime in my first pregnancy, I found that I had no time to nap or rest during the day. A teacher's workload never seems to diminish—there are always classes to prepare, and homework, essays, and exams to mark. I started going to bed very early and, on one occasion, I even had to excuse myself from one of our own dinner parties to avoid falling asleep at the table! Good friends don't mind continuing without you and letting themselves out! The moral here? Rest when you can and whenever you feel the need.

If you are independently minded (as I am), you might like doing things your way. But it is important to allow people to help you sometimes—a concept that my fiercely independent three-year-old son is slowly coming to terms with! If people offer to help around the house, in the garden, and so on, or to undertake some onerous and physically laborious task (such as painting a nursery), it is a good idea to allow these people to help. It will save you time and energy and, in the case of heavy lifting and moving, it might save you possible injury. Be sensible and conserve your energy.

The benefits of walking

During my pregnancies it also seemed as if I never had a spare moment to myself. However, I found that walking, as well as keeping me fit, gave me a chance to think and relax.

Walking is an excellent gentle form of exercise. All you need is a comfortable pair of shoes and off you go! After your baby is born, walking might again be one of the easiest ways for you to get exercise. Bundle your baby into a pram or stroller and you can stretch your legs and get fit at your own pace. Your baby will probably fall asleep or be entertained by the passing scenery. Baby backpacks are also great for older babies, especially if you're walking 'off road'. An American friend of mine takes her baby and backpack to the gym, and uses the treadmills—a handy idea if your little one doesn't like crèche or has separation anxiety. It also adds a few extra kilograms to your load and makes exercising more effective.

Feeling comfortable

Another important aspect of practice is that you become mentally comfortable doing these exercises. Practising the labour positions especially will mean that they become second nature to you and that you will be able to move in and out of different positions automatically, changing from one to the other with relative ease. During your delivery, allowing your body to move where it wants to move is important.

During her labour one friend of mine was advised that she would be more comfortable lying on a bed, although I think it was mainly the doctor's level of comfort that was being considered! However, she was firm in her requests to continue moving around—from the shower to a low stool and back again. She eventually delivered a healthy baby boy in a supported squat position and felt an incredible connection to what she described as the 'earth goddess'.

Even if this is not your scene, the message here is simple—the most important thing is being comfortable in your skin and knowing your own mind. This, coupled with physical movements that have become second nature to you, will empower you, help you to remain physically strong and flexible during your pregnancy, and help you to prepare for labour. Obviously you must consider the advice of your medical practitioner, but don't allow yourself to be coerced into unnecessary treatments that you are not happy about.

Planning for labour

If you want to experience the labour you plan, it is important to know what you want, and to ensure that your birthing partners know your wishes. It is also important for you to discuss your birth plans with your medical practitioner before you go into labour. Jot these ideas down and ensure that you are explicit about your wants and needs. It is also a good idea to include the dreaded 'what ifs?'. You should discuss alternative plans with your birthing partners, and explore the kind of care that you want to receive if your labour becomes complicated. Your written birth plan can then be referred to at any point by you and your medical staff.

If you choose to give birth away from home, visit your chosen birthing centre or delivery suite beforehand, and see what kinds of props are available for your use. Think about the kinds of extra things that you might want to bring with you, and have them packed in advance.

Every person is an individual

Every woman is different and each pregnancy is different. I was comfortable continuing with strong backwards bending, right into my final trimester. In contrast, one of our *P&F* instructors in Scotland, who is much more flexible than I am, found backwards bending extremely uncomfortable and ruled it out of her regular practice. Although I continued backwards bending, I avoided very strong hip stretches—which would have played havoc with my sacroiliac joints.

One of my students has a difference in leg lengths as a result of congenital hip dysplasia, and experiences very little movement through her hips and pelvis. During her pregnancy she experienced greater hip movement than ever as a result of the effect of relaxin in her system, helped by her regular stretching of the affected area. Her particular priority was the hip flexors (muscles that lift the thighs forwards) and adductors (muscles that bring the thighs together).

Regardless of how diligent you are in your practice, there will probably come a time when you simply cannot perform some exercises because you are physically limited by your size and shape. One of the greatest sources of frustration for me was my eventual inability to put on a pair of socks gracefully and easily! I also missed being able to sleep on my stomach. Even from very early in my pregnancies my breasts felt very uncomfortable in this position.

All of these things, however, are minor irritations and will pass quickly enough. It's best, as always, to concentrate on the more positive aspects of your pregnancy.

Let us turn to the exercises.

Chapter 1 Prenatal Exercises

Strengthening movements

1. To begin, ankle stretches

These exercises stretch your ankle joints and calf muscles. Ankle stretching is important because all the strengthening exercises we use in this book require flexibility in your ankles, and some of the most effective birth positions require the same flexibility.

Face the wall with your arms extended in front of you touching the wall, and take a pace backwards, as in the first photograph.

Lean your weight through your back leg to hold your heel on the ground. This makes the exercise most effective. Check your foot position. Your toes must be under your knee. Move the weight to the little-toe side of your foot to stop your ankle rolling inwards. (The correct foot and ankle position is shown in the last photograph.)

Now, supporting yourself on your hands, make sure your back leg is straight. Move your hips towards the wall until sufficient stretch is felt, between the knee and heel of your back leg.

To ease the stretch, move your hips away from the wall. Repeat the exercise on your other leg.

Jennifer says:

As my calf muscles tightened up during my pregnancy, I found this exercise particularly useful.

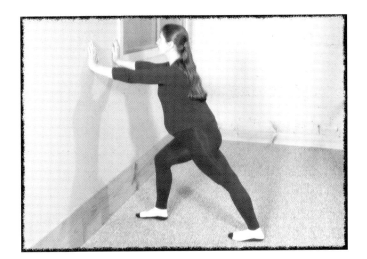

Cues

Make sure foot is under knee

Press little-toe side into floor

Press back leg straight

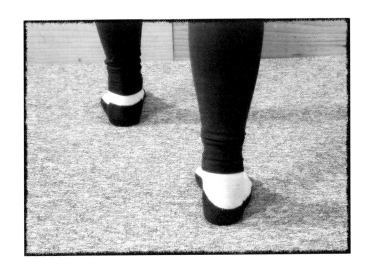

To increase the stretch effect in the calf muscle

For increased benefit you can use the *Contract–Relax* (*C–R*) technique with this exercise.

Place your weight on your back leg as for the first part of the exercise. While keeping your heel on the floor, press the ball of your foot gently into the floor and hold this effort for a count of five. (The best way to do this is to count backwards from five.) This is the *contract* part of the exercise.

To achieve the *restretch* (or what we call the *relax* component of *C–R*), breathe in, relax your leg and, as you breathe out, gently move your hips towards the wall. This alters the angle between your back foot and your leg, thereby increasing the stretch. Hold this new position for five to ten breaths. Most people will feel a strong increase in the stretch behind the knee and in the top part of the calf muscle.

To come out of this position, take more weight on your hands and gently bring your hips back from the wall. Change legs and repeat the exercise.

To increase the stretch effect in the ankle

Position your legs as for the first part of the exercise, but this time bend your back leg. Move your hips to the wall, while keeping your heel on the ground. This gives maximum flexion to your ankle joint.

For a *C–R* stretch, once in position, gently press the ball of your foot into the floor. To *restretch*, breathe in, relax your lower leg, and move your hips closer to the wall. You might feel a compression sensation in the front of your ankle joint. This is not a problem and it will disappear as soon as you come out of the exercise. Remember to stretch both legs.

For most people, the maximum ankle flexion in these two exercises will occur when the knee is bent.

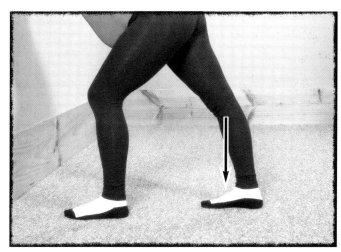

Contraction direction

Cues

C–R:
Press ball of foot
into floor

Restretch: lean further
into wall

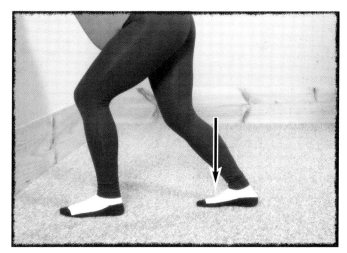

Contraction direction

2. Squats with support

Strength and flexibility in your hip and thigh area will enhance your chances of an easier childbirth. The next two exercises are the premier exercises for strengthening the muscles in your legs, hips, and lower back. They are also excellent stretching exercises and, as you sink into the squat position, you will find that your hip ligaments, buttock muscles, part of your hamstring muscles, and your ankles are being effectively stretched.

A chair for support and a board (or suitable books) to go underneath your heels are needed for this exercise. The board is to stop you feeling as though you might topple over backwards as you practise. As your ankle flexibility increases, you might not need the board, but hold the chair for support to test yourself first.

Stand facing the chair with your heels on the board. Your body should be almost upright (this is the reason for the board) and your head should be in a relaxed position above your shoulders.

Stand with your feet roughly a hip-width apart. As you squat down, observe the movement of your knees. The knees must remain above the feet in the movement, and the knees must not move inwards or outwards as you move up and down.

Breathe in and, holding your breath, slowly bend your knees. Keeping your back straight, squat down as far as you can without the shape of your back changing. Rest for an instant or two in this bottom position, feeling the stretch (and how much work your legs are doing!).

Breathing out, slowly come back up using only your leg muscles. Repeat the exercise five times to begin with.

Don't be surprised to find yourself getting out of breath after only five or ten repetitions of this exercise. Working up, in time, to twenty repetitions is worthwhile.

Jennifer says:

This is good to practise—not only for labour, and to help strengthen your legs, but also to get used to lifting safely as your pregnancy advances.

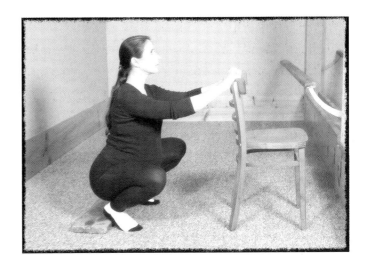

Cues

Keep heels on floor

Move up and down smoothly

Breathe in before
squatting down

Pause briefly, then
breathe out as you rise

3. Wide-angle parallel squats with support

This exercise stretches and strengthens the same muscles as Exercise 2 but, in addition, has a strong stretch effect on the muscles of your inner thigh, the adductors.

You might not be able to get your knees as wide apart as Jennifer can, so don't force your knees apart unnecessarily in trying to imitate her form. Experiment to find the right angle for you.

Good form requires your feet to be under your knees and pointing in the same direction. In addition, your knees must not travel inwards or outwards during the movement.

Hold the back of the chair, and slowly let your hips sink down as low as you can, *under control.* You will find that you won't be able to sink as deeply with your legs and your feet in this position.

Lower yourself down gently and slowly into your full squat position, pause there for an instant, and use the strength of your legs to lift yourself out to the start position.

Try for five repetitions at first and, as you become stronger, ten or more. You might consider your legs adequately strong if you can do twenty repetitions of Exercise 2 and then, after a short break to regain your breath, twenty repetitions of Exercise 3. Of course, as your pregnancy advances, fewer will be needed to provide an adequate effect.

Jennifer says:

This is a great strengthening exercise, but a lot of hard work. Start in a comfortable position and don't overdo it.

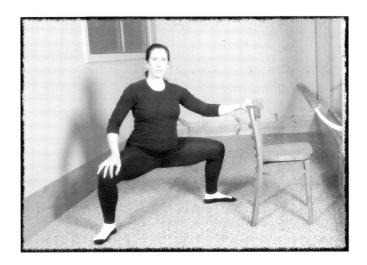

Cues

Feet under knees

Feet flat on the floor

Use legs not arms!

Breathe in to begin

Pause briefly in bottom position

Breathe out as you lift up

4. The imaginary chair

Looking at the photograph will give you all the instructions you need to do this exercise effectively. Take off your socks to increase your grip on the floor. Position a chair alongside you for assistance if necessary.

Lean with your back up against a wall and your feet far enough away from the wall so that when you are in the position that Jennifer is demonstrating, your feet will be underneath your knees.

Slowly wriggle down the wall until your thighs are roughly parallel with the floor. Until you try this exercise, you will not realise just how difficult it is to hold your weight up with your knees bent at 90 degrees. To begin with, hold the position for ten seconds or so, and plan on gradually working up to thirty seconds—or even a minute.

Use the chair alongside you to help lift yourself out of the position by using your arm.

Warming-up your body in this way will make your body much more limber for the stretching exercises.

Jennifer says:

This is a lot harder than it looks.

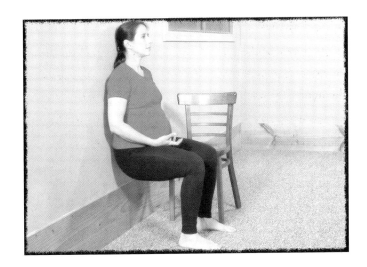

Cues

Feet under knees

Thighs parallel with floor

Use support to stand up

How to pick things up from the floor

The first photographs shows how *not* to pick something up from the floor! Notice the following problems.

- Jennifer's weight is on her left leg.
- She is bending her back and her hips.
- She is leaning to the side to pick up the footstool in front of her.

This is all inefficient, with the possibility of pulling a muscle in your lower back, or worse. In addition, as you become increasingly pregnant, you will find that the tendency to overbalance in this sort of movement is increased.

The second photograph shows the recommended technique.

- Keep your weight evenly over both feet.
- Hold the object close to the body (if it is heavy, hold with *straight* arms).
- Try to keep your whole body balanced and use your whole body in the movement.
- Bend your knees to minimise bending forwards from your hips.
- Whatever angle your body makes with the floor, hold your trunk as straight as you can.
- Take in a breath and hold the breath while doing the actual lifting.
- Use your legs to do the lifting!

If you watch young children bend down to pick up things, you will notice that this is exactly the way that they lift. (In time, of course, they learn to lift things badly, like the rest of us!)

Jennifer says:

Practise, practise, practise!

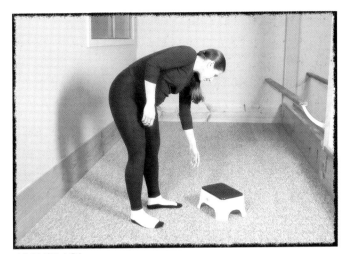

WRONG!

Cues

Face object to be lifted

Bend knees

Minimise bending forwards

Hold trunk straight

Weight evenly distributed

Hold close to body

Take in a breath before lifting

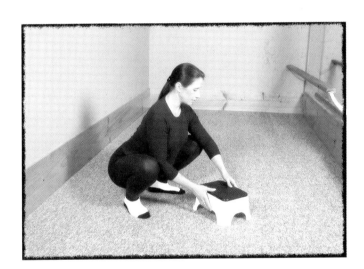

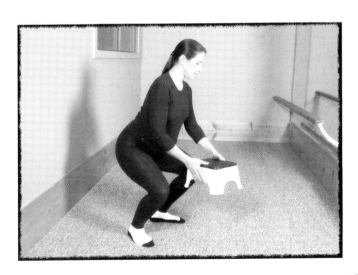

Flexibility exercises

5. Chair forwards bend, with and without support

This next exercise is one of the best movements to stretch tight lower-back muscles—muscles that often become tight during pregnancy. As the pregnancy advances, your pelvis tilts forwards, and the lower-back muscles become tighter.

Sit on the front edge of the chair as shown, hands on knees for support. Lower yourself into the stretch position *using the strength of your arms alone.* Avoid using your lower-back and upper-back muscles to support yourself in any way at all.

Let your body slump, controlling the movement with your arms. Go as far forwards as you can with your hands on your knees.

Look at the second photograph. Jennifer has placed a low footstool in front of her to be used as a support. She is resting all her upper body weight on both hands with her elbows slightly bent and her head hanging forwards in a relaxed position. Make sure that you breathe rhythmically and deeply, trying to let your entire body relax.

You can control the degree of stretch completely by the extent to which you let your arms bend. Try to remain in your final stretch position for five to ten breaths.

The last photograph shows the strongest stretch position, but if you get enough stretch using a support, use one!

To come out of the stretch position, reverse the order. *Ensure that you are lifting yourself up by your arms, one at a time!* The most common mistake is to lift up using your back muscles.

You might find that doing the exercise a second time gives you an even better stretch than doing it the first time, because your muscles have warmed-up. More importantly, your body has become used to the sensation of being in the position. In most exercises, you will find that a second attempt will yield a better stretch position, so make this your standard way of working.

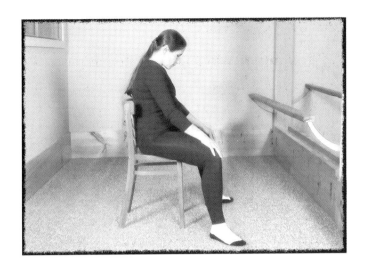

Cues

Lean on arms at all times

Hold knees for support

Lower yourself with arms

Breathe!

Use a support if necessary

Lift yourself to start position using arms

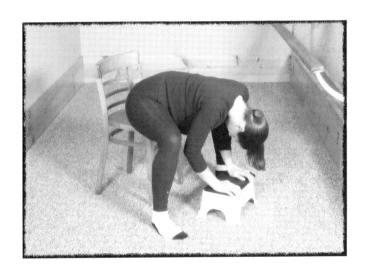

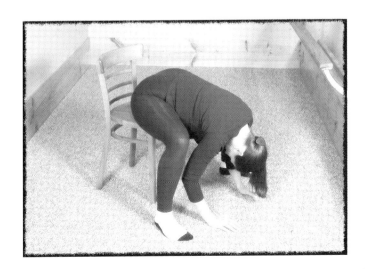

6. Chair side bend

The starting position of this exercise is the same as for the exercise you have just done. Sit on the front edge of your chair, using your hands on your knees for support. Lean to one side, letting that elbow bend, until you are leaning on it, and let your head go to the side also. Let yourself down into as strong a stretch position as you can handle. If you find that leaning on your elbow stretches you too much, you can put a pillow in between your waist and the leg that you are leaning towards.

If you wish to intensify the stretch, reach your arm out above you as shown in the second photograph.

The third photograph in the sequence shows Jennifer in an even more strongly stretched position, where the back of her shoulder is being used as support, in addition to her holding the front of the seat. She has also introduced a rotation into the movement, by looking up towards the ceiling.

You can move the stretch from the side of your waist deeper into your lower back by letting your top shoulder roll forwards (towards your toes). Make these movements slow, because very small changes in the position of your shoulder can make big differences in the stretch in your waist.

Roll your shoulder further forwards to relieve the stretch; use that arm to lift yourself back up.

Stretch the other side. Don't be surprised if they are different. Next time you stretch begin with the tighter side. The general principle is that you should stretch the tighter side, then stretch the looser side, and then stretch the tight side again.

See Exercise 26 for a stronger version.

Jennifer says:

A nice, gentle exercise for your waist and lower back—with no hamstring stretch.

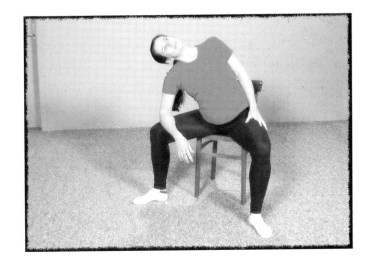

Cues

Lean on arm at all times

You can hold the seat
for support

Reach top arm out

Breathe!

Roll top shoulder forwards
to move stretch

Lift yourself to start position
using arms

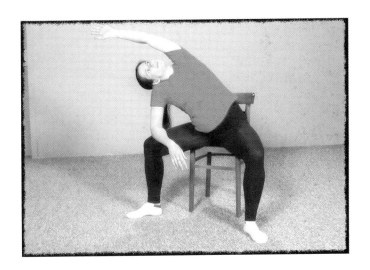

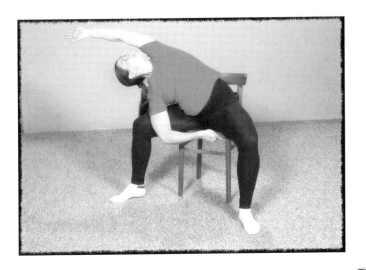

Standing version

The next photographs show the exercise done in a standing position, using the chair as support. The main difference is that the standing version also stretches some of the muscles of your hip as well as the muscles of your waist. Make sure that you lean on a secure chair or bench.

Lean to the side as far as possible *before* extending your top arm. This is because the initial position might be strong enough, and because this order of movement is safer. Stretch both sides.

Jennifer says:

Make sure your support is really stable.

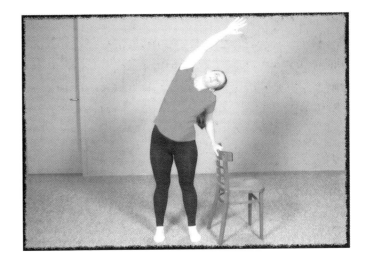

Cues

Lean on support

Lean to the side as far as you can

Reach out top arm

Breathe!

Roll shoulder forwards to move stretch

Bend legs to stand up

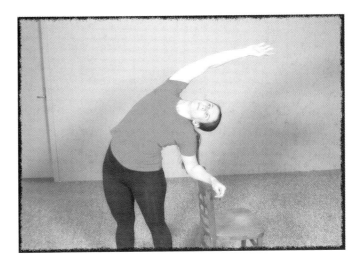

7. Chair upright rotation

As your pregnancy progresses, you will find that movements that rotate your spine become increasingly difficult—if only because of the sheer volume of the foetus growing inside you. Nonetheless, these are the very movements that can make your body feel very comfortable.

Using a chair provides the most effective means of doing these exercises effectively and safely.

Sit *across* a chair so that one leg is bearing against the back of the chair. Hold the back of the chair with both hands as shown, and use your arm strength to turn your shoulders gently away from the leg that is bearing against the chair.

Breathe in before you do the movement; and perform the rotation as you breathe out. Hold the stretch for three to five breaths in and out, and then release yourself.

Turn around on the chair and repeat all directions for the other side.

The second photograph shows a more advanced hand position.

The last photograph shows exactly where you can expect to feel the stretch—in the middle and upper back.

Do the exercise on both sides to determine which is your tighter side, and begin with this tighter side the next time that you do the exercise.

A *contraction* can improve your rotational flexibility dramatically. Once in the final stretch position take in a breath and brace yourself. Use your waist muscles to try to twist yourself gently back out of the position.

After you perform the contraction, breathe out and let the body relax. Breathe in and, on a second breath out, use the strength of your arms to try to take your shoulders further around in the stretch direction.

Quite dramatic improvements in rotation can occur after doing a contraction. Improvements of 10–15 degrees are not uncommon.

Jennifer says:

One of the few 'do-able' rotations as your pregnancy progresses—and it really gets into those tight spots in between your shoulder blades.

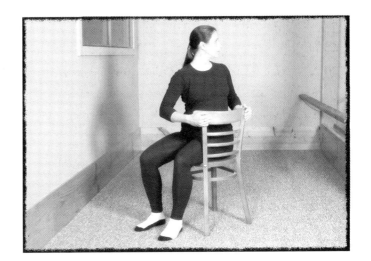

Cues

Sit with leg against seat back

Sit up straight

Grasp chair back with hands

Breathe in

On breath out, twist to side

Stretch both sides

C–R:
Try, very gently, to twist out of position

Restretch on breath out: try to twist further

Do the other side

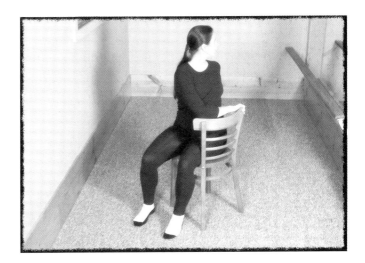

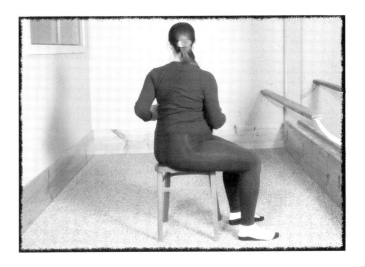

8. Gentle floor rotation

This is one that can be done anytime; all you need is a floor.

Sit with your bent legs in front of you, and place an outstretched arm on the floor behind you (as shown in the first photograph). Try to have your hand as close to the middle of your body as you can. Reach your other arm across to the outside of your knee.

Take in a breath. As you breathe out, use the arm you are leaning on and the arm braced on the knee to twist your shoulders around gently until you feel a pleasing stretch. This might be in the middle or lower back, or in both. Hold the stretch for a few breaths in and out.

Stretch the other side.

A *contraction* can help loosen tight muscles. Once in a stretch position, breathe in, brace yourself (lift your chest to make sure that your back is straight) and *try* to twist out of the position. Use a modest effort. Stop, breathe in and, while breathing out, use the strength of your arms to go a little further, gently, in the stretch direction.

The second photograph shows an alternative support position. Try both and see which you prefer.

Jennifer says:

I like to do this before going to bed—gentle and easy.

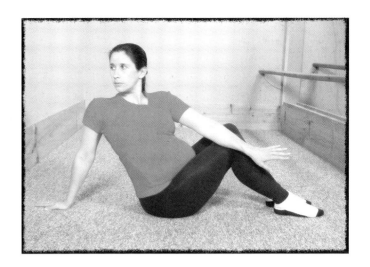

Cues

Lean on arm

Other arm outside knee

Straight back

Breathe!

C–R:

Brace; gently try to twist back

Restretch: breathe out;
try to go further

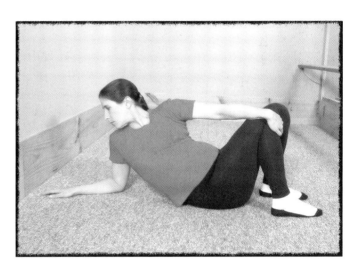

Showing the pelvic tilt on a chair

Maintaining full pelvic movement forwards and backwards will assist you in giving birth. It will also help your back to feel comfortable in the later stages of pregnancy.

The photographs show the extent of the movement Jennifer had a few weeks before giving birth. Notice that there was little movement of her pelvis backwards.

To practise, sit towards the front edge of your chair, with your feet underneath your knees and your feet flat on the floor.

With your hands on your knees, gently arch your back backwards and feel your body's weight come further forwards onto your bottom bones. In the process, your lower-back muscles will tighten up.

The second photograph shows the reverse movement. Two factors limit the rearward tilt of your pelvis at this stage:

- the volume of the foetus in front of your spine and between your abdominal wall and the ribs; and
- tightness in your lower-back muscles.

Tilting your pelvis is a gentle exercise for your lower back and feels very nice to do.

Positioning your pelvis backwards or forwards can also have specific effects in different exercises. In the next exercise, for example, rolling your pelvis forwards will increase the intensity of the exercise significantly. In later exercises, rolling your pelvis backwards will allow stretching of muscles such as your hip flexors (the muscles that lift your leg towards your chest) and and the front muscles of your thigh.

In addition to these effects, research suggests that rocking your pelvis backwards and forwards gently helps the discs of your spine to retain their fluid content, which maintains them at maximum thickness and height.

Jennifer says:

This will give you a gentle lower-back stretch, and it will help you to become more aware of your posture.

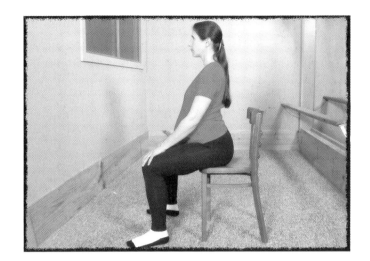

Cues

Gently arch spine;
roll hips forward

Gently contract abdominal
muscles; roll hips back

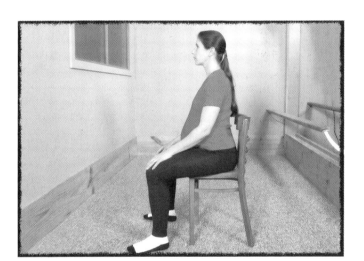

9. Chair *piriformis*

Piriformis is a small muscle deep in your hip. If it is tight, *piriformis* can cause a variety of problems in pregnancy, including pain in your hip, stiffness in your lower back, and sciatica. In severe instances, *piriformis* syndrome has been known to mimic the effects of disc impingement, giving rise to severe sciatica and referred pain in different parts of the hips, legs, and feet. It is important to keep *piriformis* supple.

Sit with your ankle on your knee and your foot underneath the knee for a stable support, as shown in the first photograph. The second photograph shows this aspect from the side. For some people, just putting the ankle on the knee in this way will give a useful stretch in the hip.

To make the stretch stronger, lean forwards from your waist towards the top foot while maintaining your spine straight or even slightly hollow, as shown in the third photograph. Rest in this stretch position for five breaths or so.

A *contraction* can make a great deal of difference in this exercise. For a count of five, press the foot resting on your knee down into your leg using the muscles of your hip. Stop pressing, take in a breath and, on a breath out (and while supporting yourself with your hands as shown), lean a little further forwards until the required stretch is felt in your hip. Hold the final stretch position for five to ten breaths. Don't forget to do both sides.

To bring yourself out of the final position, lift yourself out with your arms (but not using the muscles of your legs and your hips).

Jennifer says:

Simply a fantastic and effective exercise that requires no strength or balance.

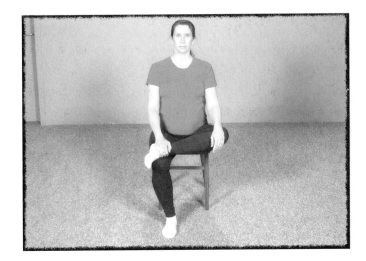

Cues

Foot underneath knee on support leg

Other ankle on knee

Keep trunk straight

Lean forwards over ankle

C–R:

Press foot towards floor

Restretch: take a breath in; lean further forwards

Use arms to recover

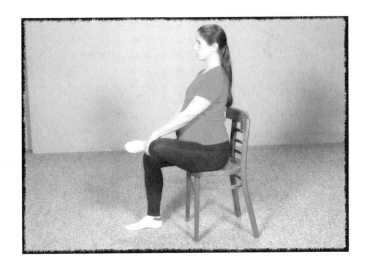

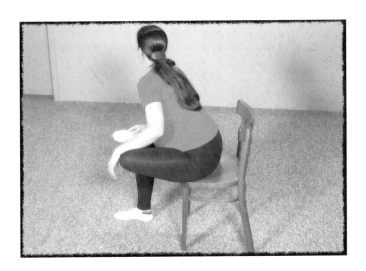

10. Floor kneeling forwards and backwards bend ('angry cat' pose)

This is a very simple but effective stretch that feels lovely to do. If you are a cat owner, you might notice that this resembles one of the few stretching exercises they do.

Kneel on all fours with your hands underneath your shoulders and your knees underneath your hips. Hold your head in a neutral position. Arch your back and take your head back as far as you can—as Jennifer is demonstrating in the first photograph. This action contracts all the muscles of your lumbar spine from the neck through to the lower back.

Next, slowly drop your head forwards and, by gently tightening your tummy muscles, bend your spine forwards in the opposite direction. All the muscles of your spine are given a gentle stretch.

This exercise gently moves your spine forwards and backwards through its full range of movement.

Gentle *contractions* can improve the results.

In the first position, gently try to draw your hands towards your knees, as though you were trying to slide them along the floor but without letting them move.

In the second position, gently try to push your hands and knees away from your body at the same time. This will increase the intensity of the stretch in your middle and upper back quite significantly.

Perform a number of these sequences. Start by doing the exercise a number of times forwards and backwards without contractions. Then add contractions for another repetition or two.

End the exercise with the forwards-bending position (see the second photograph), without contractions, to relax your body as completely as possible.

Jennifer says:

Fantastic! One of the few achievable backwards bends as your pregnancy progresses. Also good to practise if your baby is a posterior presentation, because it is said to encourage the baby to move into the best position for birth.

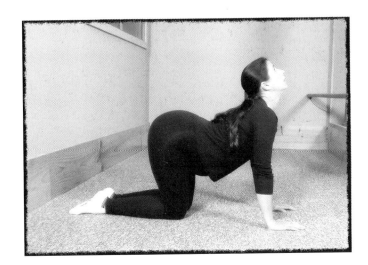

Cues

Hands under shoulders;
knees under hips

Lift head up and arch back

To increase stretch,
pull hands to knees

Relax body

Tighten tummy;
curl head to chest

To increase stretch
push hands away

Finish by curling forwards

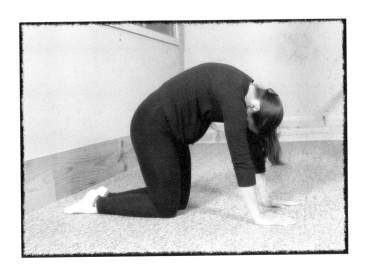

11. Floor relaxed lunge

As pregnancy advances, your pelvis tilts further forwards. One consequence is that some of the superficial and deep muscles of your hips (the hip flexors) adjust their length to their new position, becoming tighter than normal. Postpartum, these shorter muscles can resist your pelvis returning to its former position. This can be one of the major causes of lower-back pain following giving birth. Keep these muscles as supple as possible using the following exercise.

Kneel down and extend one leg out behind you while keeping the other in front of you as shown in the first photograph. Use a support under your hands if you cannot place them on the floor easily. If you wish, use a pillow under your back knee for comfort. Support your weight on your hands, breathe deeply, and let the weight of your body draw the hips forwards and down towards the floor.

Don't try to stretch these muscles too strongly. The effect of gravity alone will be enough to provide a sufficient stretch. Hold the final position for five breaths.

As with the previous exercise, you can intensify the stretch by trying to draw your hands gently towards your back knee while lifting your chest forwards and upwards.

To come out of the stretch, relax your muscles completely, change your legs over, and repeat all directions for the other side.

A *contraction* can loosen tight muscles. In the stretch position, *gently* try to press your back knee into the floor, for a count of five. If this action does not have the desired effect, think about gently pulling your back leg *forwards*. Relax and let the weight of your body provide the extra movement.

As with all exercises, you might find a significant improvement if you run through the exercise a second time. Chapter 3 will provide you with a stronger version of this exercise if you require—but for most people the version just described will be a sufficient stretch, *if* you let yourself relax into it for enough time.

Jennifer says:

An excellent exercise that I designed when stronger versions no longer suited me. You might find it very strong, but make an effort to relax. You will find the C–Rs particularly effective.

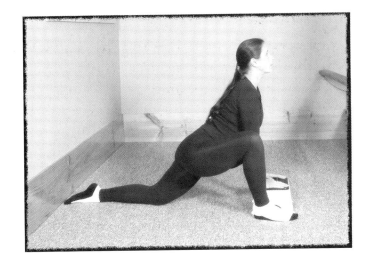

Cues

Front foot under knee

Stretch out back leg

Let gravity do all the work

To increase stretch,
pull hands back

C–R:
Press back knee into floor

Restretch: sink closer to floor

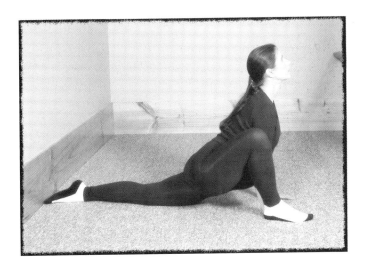

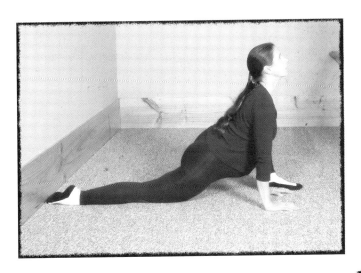

12. Wall and floor *piriformis*

This exercise provides a variation to Exercise 9 (chair *piriformis*), and is one that allows the final position to be held comfortably for a considerable time.

Position yourself a suitable distance away from the wall, fold one leg over the knee of the other as shown, and move the foot of your other leg down the wall enough to provide a stretch in your hip.

Moving your foot down the wall will increase the stretch in your other hip.

The second photograph shows one way of making the exercise stronger and more effective. Jennifer has placed one hand on the knee of the leg that is closer to her and pushed that knee away from her.

If you wish to loosen the *piriformis* muscle of this hip further, a *contraction* can be used. Press the foot of the leg resting on the knee into your thigh for a count of five.

Relax, take a breath in, and *restretch.* The restretch can be applied in two ways. The first way is to press the knee further away from you. The second way is to slide your foot further down the wall to tighten up the position. Do not let your hips and lower back come off the floor—letting your back bend defeats the stretch.

The final photograph shows a stronger position. By having her bottom closer to the wall and by sliding her foot down the wall from this position, Jennifer makes the stretch much stronger. Do not be in too much of a hurry to get into this position!

Once you have stretched one side, repeat all directions for the other side.

Jennifer says:

There is little effort involved here because your back is completely relaxed. Try Exercise 9 if there is too much pressure on the base of the spine.

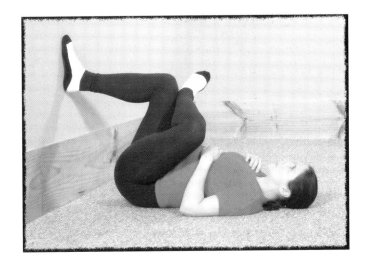

Cues

Slide foot down wall
to tighten stretch

C–R:
Press foot into knee

Restretch: foot further
down wall

Keep lower back and hips
on floor

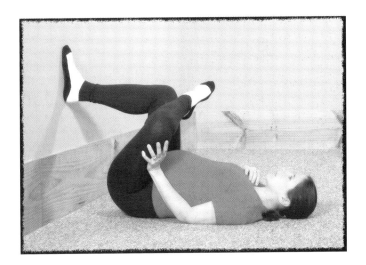

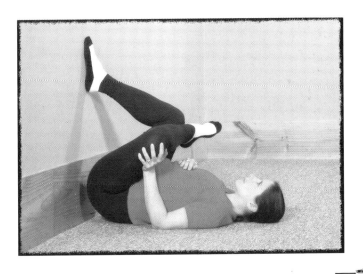

13. Back roundout (diamond pose); floor version

The purpose of both versions of this exercise is to stretch the muscles that extend (straighten) your spine. It is very useful when the bulk of the developing foetus makes other exercises difficult. By combining two actions (lifting up against your feet and pulling forwards with your arms), any part of your back can be stretched—from the top of your neck all the way down to the base of your spine.

The three photographs show the basic form of the exercise, but there is an infinite number of positions in between. Play with the movements to find the ones that feel best for you.

Sit on the floor comfortably with your knees spread apart and your feet close enough to your body to make an angle of approximately 90 degrees at your knee joints. Move your feet a little closer or further away to relieve any discomfort in your hips; if your hips feel uncomfortable you will not be able to feel the sensations in your spine.

Let your chin go towards your chest, and let your back slump and round naturally. Gaze at the floor about 10 cm back from your knees. Very gently draw your face towards this spot on the floor. This rounds out your spine in your upper back and in your neck. Hold this position for three to five breaths.

Now gaze at your ankles, and very gently pull your face in the direction of your *feet*. Notice that this moves the point of maximum stretch to below your shoulder blades. Hold this position again for three to five breaths.

The last photograph shows Jennifer gazing at the floor a couple of metres or so in front of her, and using her arms to pull her head very gently in this new direction. This has the effect of moving the stretch down to her lower back. Hold this position for a few breaths.

This stretch can be extremely pleasing, as the progress of pregnancy almost always makes the lower-back muscles tight.

Gentle *contractions* can be done at all points in this exercise. Once you are in a stretch position, use the muscles that are being stretched to *try* to pull your hands very gently away from your feet.

The *restretch* is done by *very, very gently* pulling your head further in the initial stretch direction. Hold for three to five breaths in and out.

Once you have finished this exercise you might care to repeat Exercise 8 (gentle floor rotation) because it has the effect of softening any muscles that might have remained tight.

Jennifer says:

An all-purpose exercise that can get any tight spot in the back. Wriggle around to find the best positions.

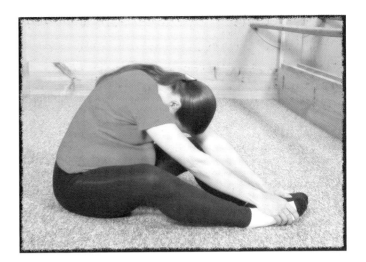

Cues

Gently pull face to floor

Pull face towards feet

Pull face in front of feet

Breathe!

C–R:

Gently pull back from hands

Restretch: gently pull further

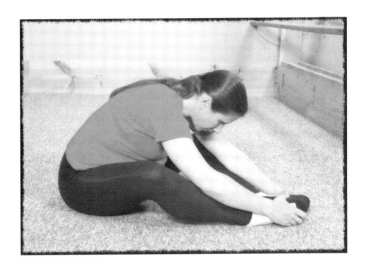

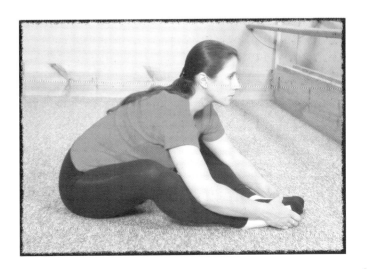

Chair version

A similar exercise can be done on a chair for convenience. The main effects of this variation will be felt in your neck and upper back.

Sit on a chair and, while supporting yourself on your hands, let your chin move forwards to your chest. Rest in this position for a moment, feeling the stretch in your neck.

Reach your hands up to the back of your head. If your neck is tight, place a couple of fingers on the back of your head. Otherwise, interlace your fingers and slowly let some of the weight of your arms rest on your head. Breathe in and out.

Let your body slump as far as is comfortable. This action moves the stretch further down your back.

A *C–R stretch* can relieve tension from this area. Holding your head, gently press back into your hands for a count of five. Stop pressing, breathe in, and, as you breathe out, cautiously apply a little extra weight to the back of your head. Hold the new position for a few breaths.

Take your hands off your head before sitting up.

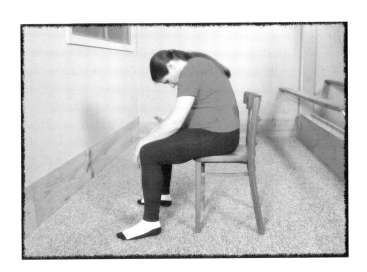

Cues

Chin to chest

Apply fingers to back of head

Breathe!

To increase stretch,
slowly slump

C–R:
Press back against fingers

Restretch: gently pull forwards

Take hands off head

Sit up

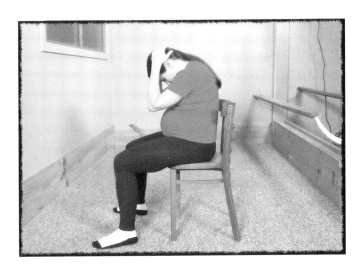

Standing pelvic tilt

The *seated* pelvic tilt was practised following Exercise 8. We are now going to practise the *standing* pelvic tilt. Being able to perform this movement guarantees success in the hip and leg exercises that follow.

In the first photograph, Jennifer has exaggerated this pelvic movement. This makes her abdomen protrude even further than normal, and her back hollows even more.

The next photograph shows the opposite movement. Here, her buttock and abdominal muscles together have been used to tilt her pelvis backwards ('tucking the tail under'). This has the effect of flattening her lumbar curve and also flattening her abdominal wall to some extent.

Stand with your weight evenly on both feet, with your legs slightly bent. Place your hands at the base of your spine if that helps you to visualise and feel the movement more effectively. Move your pelvis backwards and forwards through its full range a few times. Feel the effect that this has. Note any stretch sensations at the top of your thighs. Note which muscles you need to contract to achieve the movements.

Practising these pelvic moves is one way of making your lower back feel more comfortable. However, the reason for practising the standing pelvic tilt at this point is to learn the most effective ways to isolate stretching sensations in your hip flexors and in the large muscles at the front of your thighs. These are the focus of the next exercise.

Jennifer says:

Correct pelvic alignment will help to alleviate any pain from poor posture, especially while standing.

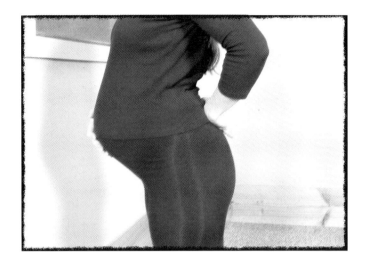

Cues

Let back arch

Feel any changes

Use buttock/abdominals to tuck the tail under

Feel stretch in front of legs

Breathe, and repeat

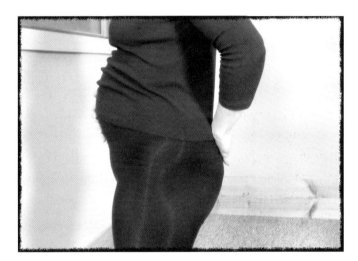

14. Standing front leg

This exercise is excellent for people who have 'problem' knees and who cannot do other thigh stretches. The intensity of this exercise can be very finely regulated and there is little compression force on your knee joints themselves.

Stand opposite a wall, supporting yourself with one arm. Hold the foot of your opposite leg with your other hand. If you can't reach your foot with your hand, use a strap or the like.

Now practise the standing pelvic tilt. While holding your foot fairly close to your bottom, use your bottom muscles to tuck your tail under. This will have two effects:

- the first is that your lumbar spine will flatten;
- the second is that you will feel a strong stretch in the front of your folded leg.

Keeping your tail tucked under, gently pull your foot as close to your bottom as you can, and hold that stretch position for a few breaths in and out.

A *contraction* can intensify the stretch significantly. There are two ways that this contraction can be done.

- The first is to try to straighten your folded leg, while you are still holding your foot. The *restretch* is to pull your foot closer to your bottom.
- The second is to draw the knee of your folded leg gently towards the wall, while resisting the movement with your buttock muscles. The *restretch* is to try to pull the folded leg gently past the straight one—to behind you if possible.

Hold the final stretch position achieved for five to ten breaths. Relax, and stretch the other side.

Don't be surprised to find a difference between your left and right thighs—this kind of asymmetry is common. However, if you do find such asymmetry, the next time that you do this exercise, start with your tight side, then do your looser side, and finish by stretching the tight side again. In time the asymmetry will be reduced.

Jennifer says:

To get the best effect from this exercise, and to do it safely, your pelvis must be in the correct position (as shown in the photo). Practise the pelvic tilt before you bring your heel to your buttock.

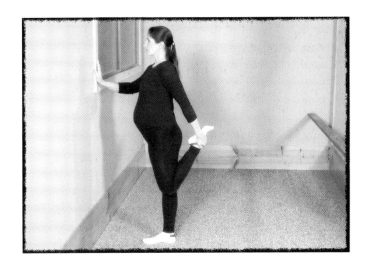

Cues

Hold foot or use strap

Tuck tail under

C–R:
Try to straighten leg

Restretch: tuck tail,
and pull foot closer

C–R:
Try to pull knee forwards

Restretch: tuck tail under,
and try to pull leg back

15. Floor-supported front thigh

An advantage of this front-thigh stretch is that it can be held without effort for considerable periods of time. Jennifer is demonstrating this exercise while sitting on a firm cushion, but any suitable support will do.

To ensure that your entire thigh is stretched, *your hips need to be level*. If you are loose enough, you can try the exercise on the floor, but make sure that both sides of your bottom are in contact with the floor. (If one hip is higher, ligaments on the inside of your folded knee can be overstretched.)

When folding your knee and pulling your foot into position alongside your hip, physically move your calf muscle out of the way to reduce the strain on your knee. Make sure that your foot points straight behind you, and that your sole faces the ceiling.

If you cannot sit like this, put a blanket under your shin, with your toes off the edge, so that your ankle does not need to be completely straight.

Just sitting in this position can be a very effective stretch for many people. Stay in the position until you feel that you have had enough stretch. Roll *away* from your folded leg and stretch the other side.

A *contraction* can improve the stretch position. Gently try to straighten your folded leg, by pushing your foot into the floor. Stop pressing, take in a breath, let your whole body relax and go soft. The weight of your body will bring your bottom closer to the floor.

To increase the stretch further, you can lean back either against a wall or onto your elbows—whichever feels comfortable and controllable. Make sure that your lower back does not bend further backwards (hyperextend) when you try this. Tucking the tail under a little will help.

To increase the stretch even further, a pelvic tilt can be done while in the final stretch position. Use your buttock muscles to tilt your pelvis backwards gently (the tail-tucking movement). Because some of the muscles of your thighs are attached to the top of your pelvis, tilting your pelvis backwards will increase the stretch in the front of your thighs significantly.

Once you finish, roll away from your folded leg to come out of the stretch—rather than lifting yourself directly forwards. This minimises the stress of the exercise on your knee and on your lower back. Make sure you stretch the other side.

Jennifer says:

If this is too strong, try Exercise 14 as a warm-up. Have a firm cushion handy.

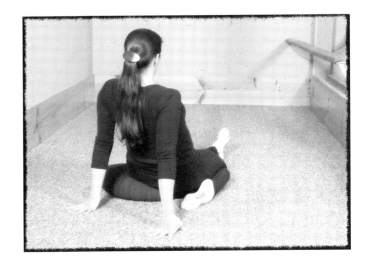

Cues

Roll calf muscle out of way

Hips must be level; use support if necessary

C–R:
Try to straighten bent leg

Restretch: lean back gently, and tuck tail under

Do not let back hyperextend

Roll away from folded leg

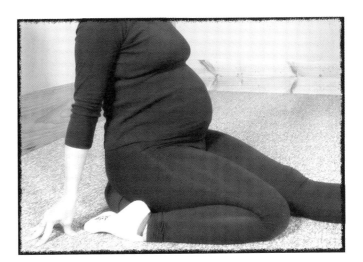

16. Standing supported forwards bend

This exercise is a gentle but effective stretch for the muscles of your hamstrings—the muscles that run from your bottom bones to below your knee, at the back of your leg. It is a good idea to stretch your calf muscles first, as a warm-up.

Stand opposite a strong kitchen chair or a bench. Have your legs separated, as shown in the top photograph, opposite. Lean forwards gently until you feel a stretch in the back of your front leg.

If the sensation is too strong, bend your front leg slightly, as Jennifer is demonstrating in the photograph below. If you are using the bent-leg version, you can increase the stretch by slowly trying to straighten your front leg. If there is too much stretch in your *back* leg, bring it forwards until the sensation disappears.

The stretch can be increased in intensity by holding your back completely straight and leaning further forwards, onto your elbows—as Jennifer is demonstrating in the second photograph.

If you are loose enough, you can attempt the third position, in which Jennifer is supporting herself on her elbows on the back of the chair.

As the weight of your body is supported in all of these positions, give your hamstring muscles a good stretch by staying in the final stretch position for at least ten breaths in and out. Lift yourself out of the stretch position by bending both legs and using your arms—rather than using the muscles at the back of your legs to help yourself up. This takes the strain away from getting out of the final stretch position. Take a breath in as you come up.

Stand up, change legs, and stretch your other side.

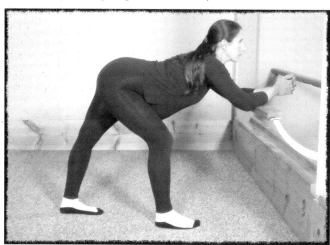

Jennifer says:

Suitable for everybody, this exercise can be as easy or as difficult as you like. Make sure you stretch your calf muscles first.

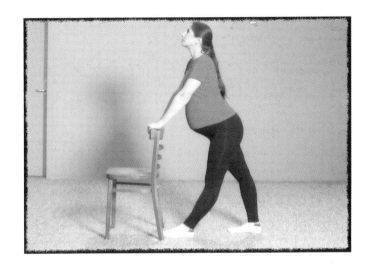

Cues

Use a sturdy support
Keep lower back straight
Lean forwards until stretch is felt
Bend front leg if required
Hold for 5–10 breaths
Use arms to recover

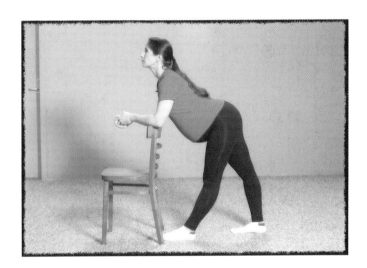

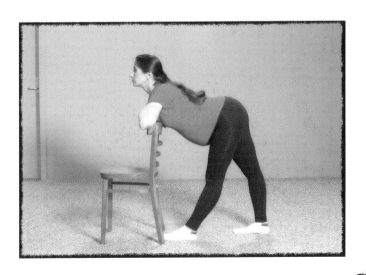

17. Standing supported forwards bend with rotation

Depending on the height of the support that you use, this exercise is much stronger than the previous one and is a combination rotation and hamstring stretch. As Jennifer is flexible, she is using a low support. You might find that using the seat of a chair is the right height support for you. Balance is easy to achieve because your body is supported.

Lean down onto the support as shown. You might lean onto the support with bent legs if you prefer, and then straighten them once in position. Lean on your hand that is on the support, letting your other arm hang down towards the floor. Lean forwards only as far as you can keep your back straight. Choose a support of a height that allows you to maintain this shape.

Take your unsupported arm out to the side while looking at it, and keep moving it further out to the side until it is as close to above you as your flexibility permits. To increase the stretch, reach your arm out above you as far as you can.

Look at the second photograph. Jennifer has extended her unsupported arm directly above her shoulder, and she is gazing past her fingertips. You can see that the top side of her chest has been opened fully, and her shoulder has been moved off her body to the maximum extent. This stretches the muscles in between her ribs, all of her abdominal muscles, and her chest and arm muscles.

Once in your final position, carefully move your hips from one side to the other, and back again. This changes the stretch in the legs, increasing the effects in the adductors.

Make sure that you breathe deeply in the final stretch position for a few breaths. Reverse the directions to get out of the stretch. Repeat for the other side.

The last photograph shows the extent to which the entire spine is given a rotation.

Bend the legs before you stand up, to take the strain off the back of the legs. If you have *a tendency to light-headedness* when standing up, take in a full breath before trying to stand, and hold the breath in until you are fully upright. This tip can be used any time that you are getting up off the floor, getting out of a seat, or standing up.

Jennifer says:

I love this exercise. Multipurpose hamstring, rotation, shoulder—this one has it all.

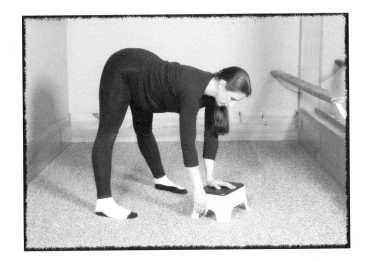

Cues

Make sure support height
is right for you

Lean forwards
with straight back

Support body on arm

Take arm to the side;
look at fingertips

Extend arm above body

To recover, bring arms together

Bend knees, and stand up

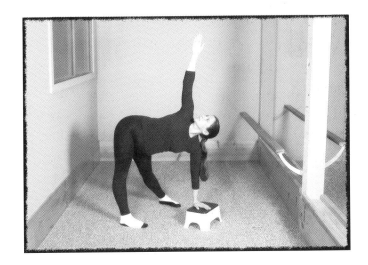

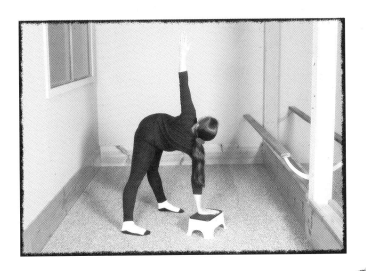

18. Floor relaxed bent knees forwards bend

This is the easiest version of the all-important hip-opening exercises that produce the flexibility crucial for easier childbirth. Everyone will be able to do a version of this exercise. This is therefore an excellent warm-up for Exercise 19—the full version of the movement.

Sit with your legs crossed as Jennifer is demonstrating in the first photograph. She is sitting with one ankle on top of the other, but there are many variations. For example:

- you might have one foot on the floor in front of the other;
- you might have your knees closer together, or further apart; or
- you can have your lower legs crossed over each other (as when sitting cross-legged).

If you find that you cannot sit on the floor in one of these positions without your back rounding, use a cushion underneath your bottom to tilt your whole body slightly forwards. This will help you to hold your spine straight without effort.

In the second photograph, Jennifer is demonstrating the leaning part of the exercise. Once you have become accustomed to sitting cross-legged with a straight back, incline your body forwards holding your back straight.

This ensures that movement of your trunk occurs as a result of your pelvis moving in between your two hip joints. This forwards-inclination movement is effective for loosening the ligaments at the front of your hip joints.

Stay in the final position for at least five to ten breaths. A longer stay in the final position has even more beneficial effects.

Jennifer says:

Next time that you are on the floor, try sitting like this. With regular practice it will become easier.

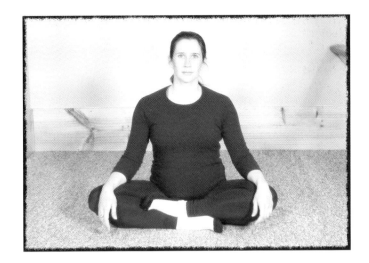

Cues

Keep trunk straight

Lean forwards only at hip joints

Hands in front for support

Breathe deeply and rhythmically

Use hands to return

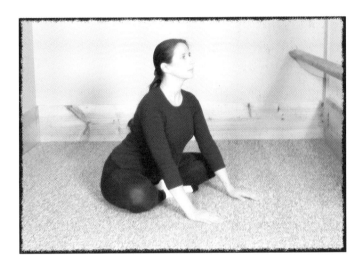

19. Wall seated knees apart plus forwards bend

This is probably one of the most important exercises for childbirth. Various support positions are shown.

In the first photograph, Jennifer is seated with her bottom up against a wall. She has a cushion underneath her hips and rolled mats to act as supports underneath her thighs. The latter supports stop the weight of her legs overstretching the muscles on the inside of her thighs.

As the weight of your legs stretches the involved muscles, you will find your legs pressing onto these supports, As this happens you can reduce the height of the support so that your legs move closer to the floor.

Once your knees are reasonably close to the floor, a forwards lean can be added. The second photograph shows Jennifer holding a support. Lift your chest up to straighten your back and then pull gently on the support to help the forwards lean. The stretch will be felt at the front of your hip joints.

The last photograph shows a more advanced position. Notice that Jennifer has leant forwards without letting her back bend at all. This ensures that the movement occurs at her *hip joints*, and not at her back! Stay in the final position for five to ten breaths.

Jennifer says:

To begin, use as many props as you need. The big secret to groin stretches is to relax. Make a conscious effort to do so. Take your time and stay in the position for a while.

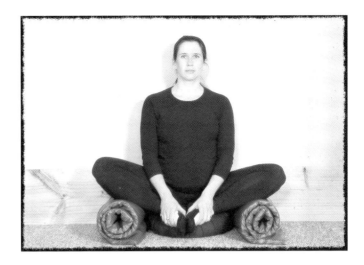

Cues

Sit on a cushion to tilt hips

Use supports under legs

Press legs into support

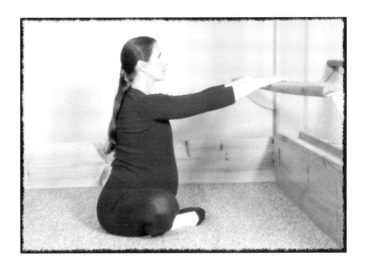

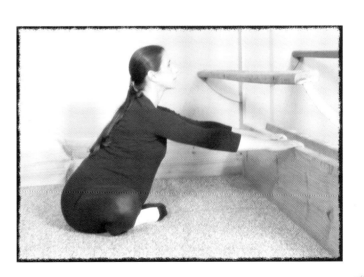

Contractions in this exercise

Contractions are extremely effective in this exercise. Lift your shoulders and place your hands on the inside of your knees and gently press your knees down towards the floor (or into the supports, if you are using them). This will stretch the muscles on the inside of your thighs. Hold this position for a few breaths.

Lift your knees up against the resistance of your arms. It is essential that you do not let your knees move even a millimetre. If this occurs, the final stretch position is reduced. Hold the contraction for a count of five.

To *restretch*, take in a breath, let the muscles of your leg relax completely (but don't let the knees move at all). On a breath out, gently push your legs further down (top photograph). If this position hurts your knees, try one of the other hip-opening exercises (Exercises 18, 21, 23, 24).

In the second photograph, Jennifer has lifted her chest to ensure that her upper back and middle back are straight, and she has her hands placed on the floor in front of her feet for support. She has leant forwards as far as she can onto her hands.

The last photograph shows the most advanced version. She has grasped her feet with her hands, and is using her strength to do two things:

- pulling her body forwards using her arms; and
- helping to hold her back straight by lifting her chest and pulling with the muscles underneath her arms.

An additional *contraction* can be done from the advanced position. Lift your chest, hold yourself in position, and use the muscles of your groin and your back to lift yourself gently away backwards from the stretch position.

Stop contracting, take in a breath, relax your hip muscles, and gently pull yourself further forwards. The sensation of this stretch is felt in the very front of your hip joints.

Hold your final stretch position for at least five to ten breaths. Your legs can be eased by straightening them, and rolling them inwards and outwards a few times.

Once you have relaxed in the *restretch* position for five to ten breaths, repeat the contractions and the *restretch* sequence once or twice more—until you feel you have stretched enough for this session.

Jennifer says:

C–Rs are particularly effective here. Do them gently. Do as many as you need to relax into a comfortable position. A good one to practise while watching television.

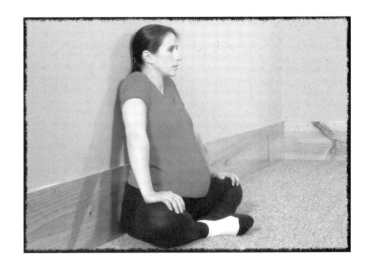

Cues

C–R:

Lift knees up against arms

Restretch: gently press legs down

Repeat C–Rs two or three times

Straighten and roll legs in and out

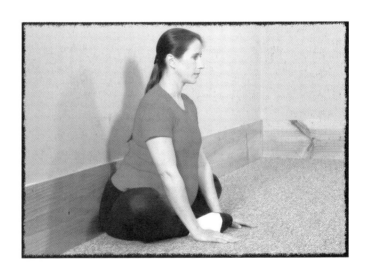

Cues (advanced position)

C–R:

Hold feet, and try to pull body back

Restretch: pull gently forwards

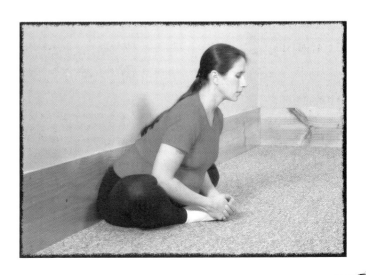

20. Chair 'sumo' rotation

Jennifer developed this exercise during her first pregnancy, because she found all the ordinary rotation poses uncomfortable in the later months. In so doing, she discovered one of *P&F*'s most powerful rotation exercises—one that can be done with effect for even the most flexible person.

Because the exercise is done from the seated position, it is suitable for somebody in an advanced stage of pregnancy. The use of your arms allows very fine control over the final rotation position.

Sit towards the front edge of your chair with your feet firmly on the floor underneath your knees as shown. Lean forwards slightly, taking your weight on your hands. If necessary, lean on a support between your feet to get into position.

Controlling your movement with your arms, lean forwards until your body is near horizontal. Lean on one arm (second photograph) and reach your other arm across to hold the ankle of the leg you are leaning on.

Press back with your hand and the arm that is on your knee, while gently pulling your bottom shoulder towards the ankle of the same leg. There should be a distinct 'push–pull' feeling.

Changes in sensation (and location) of the stretch can be made by the position of your trunk in relation to your knees. If you start the exercise with your trunk closer to the leg that you are using as your support, you will get quite different sensations from those that you will experience if you start the exercise with your trunk closer to the other leg. For best results, try a number of different positions and use the one that is most pleasing for you.

A *contraction* can improve the stretch if desired. Once in position, brace yourself and use the waist muscles to twist gently out of position for a few seconds. Breathe out and breathe in. As you breathe out again, use your arms to move you into a stronger position. *Be very gentle!*

To get out of the exercise, again take your weight on your top arm and bring your other arm up onto your other knee. Using the strength of your arms only, lift yourself out of the forwards bending position. Take a breath in before coming up. Don't forget to stretch the other side.

Jennifer says:

This one suits everybody and is 'do-able' no matter how big you are. It is one of the few rotations that you will be able to practise right up until your due date. If you think you will need a block, have one handy.

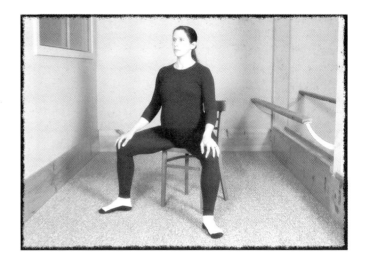

Cues

Sit on front edge of chair

Lower yourself to start

Support weight with arms

Push top shoulder back

Pull bottom shoulder to ankle

C–R:

Try to twist out of position

Restretch: go further in stretch direction

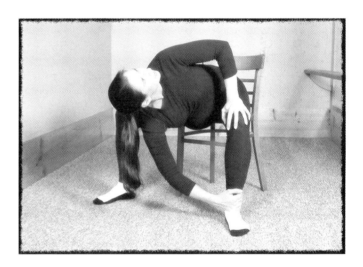

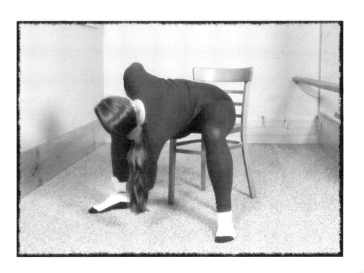

21. Knees apart folded leg forwards bend

The hip-opening action is resisted by the muscles on the inside of your thighs, and by ligaments as well. Exercise 21 moves the pelvis in between your thighs—as do Exercises 18 and 19, but with your thigh bone in a different position in relation to your hip joint. This results in a slightly different stretch.

Look at the top photograph. To get into this position, roll your calf muscles out of the way (as described in Exercise 15, floor-supported front thigh). The cushion under your hips limits the knee angle so that you don't place too much strain on your knees. If you feel any pain in your knees, don't do this exercise. Use a support of the right thickness. The tighter your leg muscles and hip joints are, the thicker the support you need to use.

Place a support in front of you. Sit with a straight back in the starting position. This will be a stretch for many people; if so, stay in this position for a few minutes.

To increase the stretch, lift your chest to ensure that your back is straight. Slowly incline your trunk forwards by letting your arms bend. Hold the position for a few breaths.

The next photograph shows a more advanced version of the pose. Jennifer has widened her knees as far as she can, and her bottom is firmly on the floor. Lean forwards with your back straight until you are leaning on your elbows.

You might not be this flexible, and might require a small support underneath your hips to take the strain from your knees. Alternatively, you might require a support in front of you to lean on.

In the final photograph, Jennifer's bottom is still in contact with the floor, her abdomen is firmly in contact with the floor, and her chest and arms are out along the floor as well. Only the very flexible will be able to get into this position.

Don't sacrifice good form to achieve what you think is a better position. Good form requires that your back be straight and that your hips stay on the ground. This ensures that your *hips* are stretched.

Don't forget that the purpose of a stretch is not to make a certain shape, but to get the stretch in the right place! Stay in your final position for at least ten breaths in and out.

Breathing deeply and rhythmically will assist your muscles to relax. You might find that getting up and walking around before trying the exercise a second or a third time will give you a greatly improved end position.

Jennifer says:

If this hurts your knees, don't do it! Substitute any of the other hip-opening exercises.

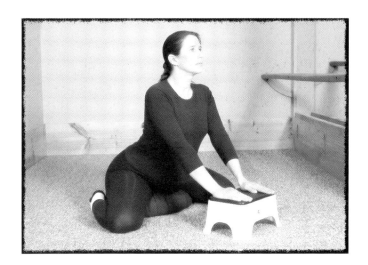

Cues

No strain in knees!
Hold back straight
Lean forwards if you can
Use arms for support
Breathe deeply and rhythmically
Use arms to recover

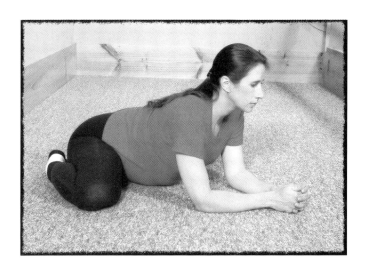

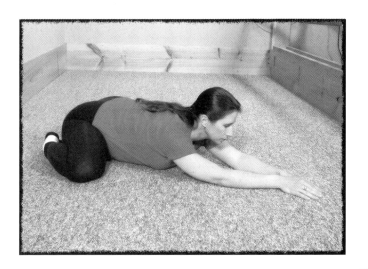

22. Floor extended-leg *piriformis*

This is the most effective stretch for your deep hip muscles. As this exercise requires suppleness in your hip flexors and front thighs, warm-up by practising Exercise 11. Look at the first photograph and imitate Jennifer's position.

Sit with one leg out in front of you and the other behind. Lean on to hip of your front leg and extend the knee to about 90 degrees, as shown in the first photograph. Place your hand behind the hip of your other leg.

The second photograph shows the essential hip-rolling action. Here, Jennifer is rolling her left hip towards her right foot, so that her hips become squarer (in relation to the line of her legs) in the action. The stretch will be felt in the hip of her folded front leg.

Rolling your hip towards your foot can be assisted by holding something out to the side (use the arm on the side you are rolling towards) and pulling yourself square. Alternatively, help your hip move by placing a hand on it, and pressing.

A *contraction* can be used in this position. Press your front foot straight down into the floor for a count of five or so. This will activate the hip muscles of your front leg.

The *restretch* is achieved by rolling your back leg hip closer to the floor.

The last photograph shows Jennifer leaning her body towards her foot from the previous position. If you are loose enough to use this second movement, make sure that the centre of your body moves in the direction of your *foot* (not your knee) for maximum effectiveness.

Stay in the final position for five to ten breaths, and then roll away from the stretch to recover. Change legs over and repeat for the other side.

A good position in this exercise is controlled by tension in *piriformis* and by how far you can extend your back leg out behind you. So, if your hip flexors and thighs are tight, you might not even be able to get into an effective first position in this exercise. If so, use Exercise 9, chair *piriformis*, instead. Alternatively, you can press the back leg into the floor as a contraction to help loosen the hip flexors.

If you are able to use Exercise 22, do Exercise 5, chair forwards bend, as a recovery movement. This is because lower-back muscles can tighten doing the floor *piriformis* exercise, a result of using your hip flexors to extend (straighten) your lumbar spine.

Jennifer says:

Although this is the most difficult of the piriformis exercises, it is really worth pursuing. If you can do it, be very strict with form. Don't worry if you can't do it yet. Take your time and work up to it.

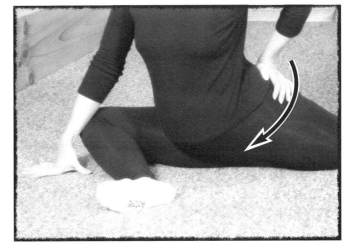

Move hip towards floor

Cues

Hip of front leg on floor

Knee of front leg at 90 degrees

Roll hip of back leg towards floor

C–R:

Press front foot down into floor

Restretch: roll back hip forwards

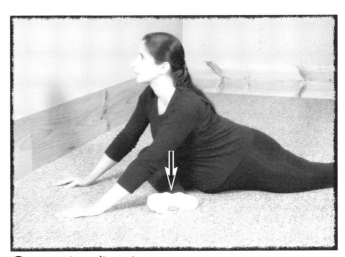

Contraction direction

Advanced:
Lean chest towards foot

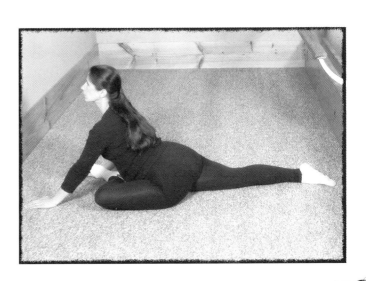

23. Wall face-up bent legs apart

Doing this exercise is simplicity itself—but don't be deceived. If the final stretch position is held for a minute or so, the stretch effect on the inside of your thighs and the hip joint itself is strong. It is excellent preparation for Exercise 24 (which follows). Look at the first photograph.

Jennifer's knees are approximately at right angles, and her lower legs are parallel to the floor. Try to achieve this position, because this will reduce the strain on your knees to a minimum.

Make sure that your entire back is in contact with the floor. In the later stages of pregnancy, you might wish to lie on a mat or a blanket to reduce the pressure on the sacroiliac area (the joints at the back of the pelvis).

The weight of your legs alone will provide a good stretch to your adductors (the inside thigh muscles) and to the ligaments at the front of your hip.

Contractions can be used by placing your hands on the inside of your knees and trying to squeeze your knees together. The *restretch* is achieved by pressing your knees a little closer to the floor.

To come out of the stretch, you might find it more comfortable to bring your knees together by using your arms—rather than by using the muscles that have been stretched. Roll to the side, breathe in, and push up with your arms.

The second photograph shows the same position—but with your head supported. You might find that having your head supported allows you to hold the final position for much longer than if unsupported. Try the exercise both ways and see which suits you.

Jennifer says:

Initially devised for one of my first pregnant students, this is a variation of a standard P&F *stretch. If it is too strong, place firm cushions under your knees to reduce the stretch.*

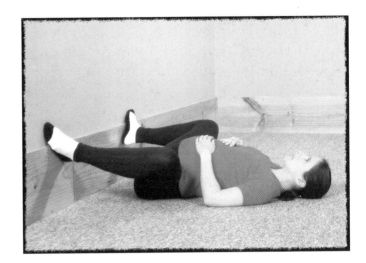

Cues

Knees make right angles

Lower legs parallel to the floor

Ensure all of spine
rests on floor

Breathe and hold position

C–R:
Squeeze knees against hands

Restretch: press legs to floor

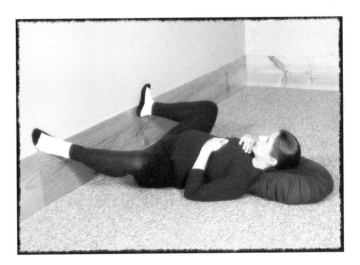

24. Wall face-up straight legs apart

This is the fundamental legs-apart exercise. Because it is done in the lying position, it can be held for a considerable time with minimal effort. Look at the photograph.

Jennifer has her hips against the wall and her whole back on the floor. Your hamstring flexibility will determine how close you can get to the wall. If you are moderately loose, you will be able to lie with your bottom up against the wall. If you are not very loose, your bottom will be a little away from the wall.

It it much better to be a small distance away from the wall, but with your hips and spine resting on the floor.

The easiest way to get into this position is to lie alongside the wall with both of your legs up the wall, and then turn yourself around so that your bottom is against the wall. Move into the stretch position to allow gravity to move your legs apart.

As with the previous exercise, do not be deceived by its simplicity. Staying in this position for four or five minutes will give you an excellent stretch. This is mainly focused in the muscles on the inside of your thighs—the muscles that pull your legs together.

You can ease the sensation on your inner thighs by bringing your legs together for a moment or two while lying in the position. When you feel ready, let gravity open your hips again. In this way, a number of repetitions can be performed without moving your body.

A *contraction* can help you get into a better final position. Place your hands on the inside of your knees, and squeeze your legs together against this resistance—for a count of five. Try not to let the legs move at all.

Restretch by pressing your legs towards the floor, or simply let gravity do the work for you. To come out of the stretch, bring your knees together by using your arms, roll to the side, breathe in, and push up with your arms.

As with the previous exercise, you might find that you get an even better effect by getting up out of the exercise position, walking around for a moment or two, and then repeating the exercise.

Jennifer says:

If the stretch is too strong on the inside of your knees, you can turn your legs in or out a little to find a more comfortable position. Pulling your toes back towards your knees adds a calf stretch and makes the stretch stronger.

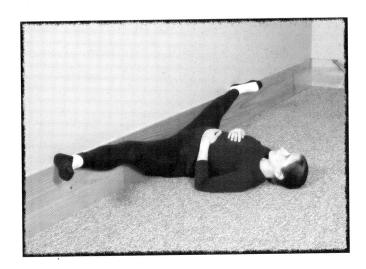

Cues

Bottom close to the wall

Whole spine on floor

Keep body relaxed

Let gravity do the work

C–R:
Hands inside knees

Try to squeeze legs together

Restretch: press legs to floor, or let gravity do the work

Breathe!

25. Floor legs apart

Derived from a basic hip-opening exercise in yoga and many other exercise forms, one of the benefits of this exercise lies in its effectiveness in stretching the muscles of your lower back and your trunk. It has a number of support positions. Look at the first photograph.

Jennifer is seated on a cushion to incline her trunk forwards a little. One leg is folded, and the other is outstretched. She has looped a strap around her foot and, to take the strain away from the hamstrings, her knee is slightly bent. She has leant her body across to her bent leg, and her elbow is placed inside her leg.

The second photograph shows a more advanced position with legs apart. Jennifer's top arm is extended as far off her body as possible, in line with her trunk. This stretches many of the biggest muscles in her back. You might find that the stretch is felt down behind your hip joint, and is very pleasing indeed.

The third photograph shows the final position if you are very flexible. Jennifer's trunk is lying against her leg, her shoulder is slightly in front of her leg, and her top arm is holding the foot. Use a strap if you wish. This is a very strong stretch for the side of your body, and is a good stretch for the hamstrings of the leg you are bending over. Whichever position you get into, hold it for at least half a minute to a minute for best effects. Breathe and try to relax.

To come out of your final position, roll your top shoulder *forwards*. As you do so you will feel the stretch move from the side of your waist further around into your back itself. If you find a position that is particularly effective for you, stay in this for a further thirty seconds or so, breathing normally.

Once you roll your shoulder far enough forwards, you will find that the stretch disappears completely. Place your top arm on the floor, and lift yourself out of the stretch position using both arms. Repeat all directions for the other side.

To finish your exercise session, use any exercise that makes your body feel comfortable and relaxed. For some, this will be a rotation exercise; for others a forwards bend.

When you are performing your final exercise, don't make any attempt to improve it in a flexibility sense. Rather, just let your body relax and feel the sensation of having had a decent stretch.

Jennifer says:

This is one of my all-time favourites. You might want to warm-up with Exercise 6 first. If you think that you need a strap, have one handy.

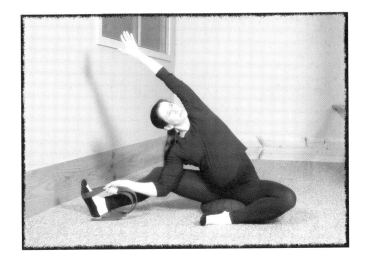

Cues

Sit on a cushion if necessary

Hold foot by strap if necessary

Bend leg if necessary

Incline trunk to side

Extend arm out above body

Roll shoulder forwards
to move stretch

Use arms to recover

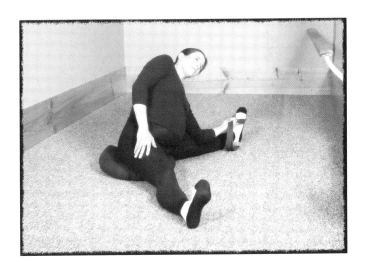

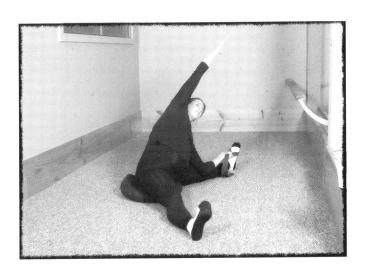

CHAPTER 2 RELAXATION

Why relaxation?

This chapter contains advice on the best relaxation and birthing positions, and an approach to acquiring the skill of relaxation. An expectant woman *needs* to be able to relax, for two critical reasons:

- to optimise her own health and the health of the unborn child; and
- to be able to give birth as easily as possible.

In the most general sense, relaxation is essential. Everyone knows this but, in a busy day, relaxation practice can be put off (and put off again!) until the day is over and the opportunity has gone. Life gets in the way of our best intentions. It is useful—perhaps even essential—for you to put aside a time for relaxation on a daily basis if possible, and this chapter presents an efficient technique for learning this skill.

Even if you are a naturally tense person, you will learn to relax properly in a couple of weeks of daily practice. This technique, a blend of old and new, has been taught to thousands of people in our classes.

However, before we begin, what are the benefits of relaxation?

The research into the processes and outcomes of developing the capacity to relax is unanimous—healing proceeds faster, potentially life-threatening conditions such as hypertension (high blood pressure) are reduced, growth and repair are accelerated, and you feel better.

Acquiring the capacity to relax is simply the best remedy to the many stressors in life. These affect our bodies through the 'fight-or-flight' syndrome which is mediated though the *sympathetic nervous system*. Relaxation accesses a parallel set of responses through the *parasympathetic nervous system*, which acts to calm many of our bodies' internal processes.

Accordingly, an expectant woman can look at relaxation in the same way as she thinks about exercise and nutrition—all are parts of a combined approach to ensure that she has done all that she can to optimise the health of her unborn child.

She can also look at relaxation as being the acquisition of a skill to facilitate childbirth itself, as Jennifer emphasised in the Introduction.

Finally, relaxation practice, as well as making you feel good at the time, will give you a reserve of wellbeing that you can use in dealing with tomorrow's problems!

So, treat yourself—put aside twenty minutes to practise and enjoy the experience.

How to use the relaxation techniques

First and foremost, use the tapes to take a well-needed break. Your body is doing a prodigious amount of work in building this new life inside you. You will certainly need to rest more often than you usually do in your normal busy daily life. But resting and relaxing are sometimes quite difficult things to do—everyone has had the experience of going to bed absolutely 'bone-tired' and not being able to rest. In contrast, after a long night of sleep (perhaps after even more hours than usual), you can wake up feeling absolutely exhausted and washed out. The reason is usually excessive brain activity and an inability to let go of the bodily tension that has built up during the day. So the first use of the relaxation tape is simply to get the brain and the body in the right state for true rest.

The *first way* to use the relaxation tape is before going to bed. Try using the relaxation tape one night, but make sure that you don't fall asleep. (Suggestions for avoiding falling asleep will be found below.) Once you hop into bed, you will notice that you fall asleep virtually immediately. And if the relaxation practice has been successful, you will wake up the next day feeling completely refreshed.

Another way to use the relaxation tape is to do the relaxation practice after you have done your other strengthening and stretching exercises. Doing this (assuming that you have the time) will leave you feeling wonderfully calm and refreshed, and will usually leave you with more energy than doing the strengthening and stretching exercises by themselves. However, if your general state is fatigued, doing the relaxation exercises can leave you feeling even *more* tired than before. This is because, during the relaxation practice, your body has a chance to relax completely—and if you are tired your body simply wants to sleep. Use this as an indication that you might need more rest generally.

The third way to use the relaxation exercise is *before* you do your stretching and strengthening exercises. Try using relaxation *before* your stretching and strengthening exercises on one day. On another day, try it *afterwards*. See which affects you the more pleasantly.

On a day when you are rushed and feeling frazzled, just do the relaxation practice. Leave the strenuous strengthening and stretching exercises for another day and simply enjoy the feeling of being completely relaxed.

Relaxation positions

An effective relaxation position is one that lets you relax, but does not encourage sleep. The following series of photographs shows Jennifer's favourite positions and use of props. The first photograph shows the recommended position for learning the technique. It allows you to feel both your stomach and chest easily. Instead of a rolled support under your knees, you can put your lower legs on a chair or couch. This is particularly effective if your legs feel heavy as your pregnancy advances. Use the other positions for variation once you are confident that you will not fall asleep.

Jennifer says:

It is really important to find a position that will enable you to relax without falling asleep. Don't practise on the bed. If you are tired, have a sleep instead!

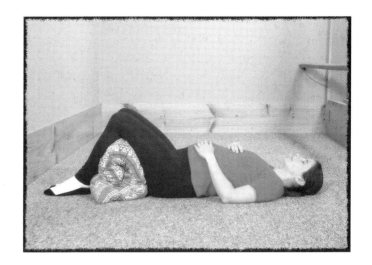

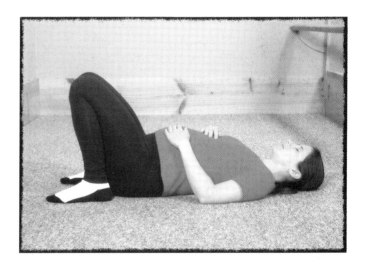

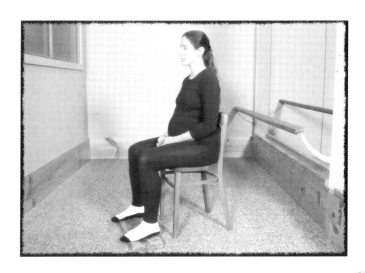

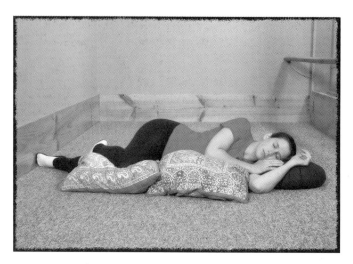

How to relax

Before we begin there are a few practical things that you need to do.

- Make sure the phone is off the hook.
- Go to the toilet.
- Wear clothing that is sufficiently warm to allow you to relax completely.
- Try to ensure that you won't be disturbed by household members for the next fifteen to twenty minutes.
- Avoid practising your relaxation exercise on your bed because the temptation to fall asleep will be very strong—even if you are trying hard to stay awake. The best relaxation is a kind of hovering between wakefulness and sleep, where you can direct the flow of your attention, but where the object of your attention does not actually disturb your state of relaxation. It is a state in which thoughts come into your mind, but in which your mind has a kind of 'watchfulness' that lets you 'observe' the thoughts without being disturbed. In its best form it is a relaxed dispassionate state.

The relaxation script

The following relaxation script (beginning on page 94) can be recorded by a friend with a nice soft voice. Play it back to yourself through headphones or a stereo. It can be used in any of the recommended relaxation positions. Depending on the reading speed, it goes for about twenty minutes or so.

The script contains various actions, some of which can be visualised if you can't physically do them. These actions are alternated with various breathing techniques.

What relaxation position should you use?

This script is best practised on the floor to begin with—because having your body's weight fully supported by the floor will allow you to do all the muscular contractions and breathing exercises most easily.

The first few times that you practise, we suggest using one of the lying relaxation positions—the one that is most comfortable for you. Jennifer commented that when she was practising, she found lying face up on a hard surface to be relatively uncomfortable for the sacroiliac joints (the joints at the back of the pelvis) in the later stages of pregnancy—the very position that was most comfortable for practice in the early stages.

You will need to use a position that is comfortable for you. As with the exercises, if your attention is distracted by some discomfort in your body you will not be able to relax properly. However, you don't want to fall asleep, and many people have told us that they have found a carpeted floor to be the ideal surface on which to practise relaxation.

As your body relaxes you will tend to feel cooler. Cover yourself with a blanket so that you don't feel cold.

Let us now go into our relaxation practice, assuming that you have chosen one of the positions in which you are lying face up.

Am I breathing properly?

Put one hand on your chest and the other on your stomach over your navel. Let your back press against the floor and your legs rest on the floor (or on a support).

Our first exercise is to learn how to breathe most effectively for relaxation. Take in a breath and see which parts of your body move. If you are breathing *abdominally* you will find that your chest does not move but that the tummy does. This is the best way to breathe if you want to relax—because breathing into your chest and lifting your shoulders are associated (by your brain) with tension and anxiety. These are the very last emotions that you want to feel if you are trying to relax.

If you find that your chest (as well as your tummy) moves up against your hand, let your whole body relax before taking the next breath in. See if you can direct the air lower down into your abdomen. If you can, you will find that only the hand on your tummy moves, and that the hand on your chest moves very little (or not at all). In time, you will find that your chest will remain completely motionless throughout the breathing exercises.

Take in a breath and feel your tummy rise under your hand. As you breathe out, feel the air leaving your body, and feel your body pressing down onto the floor.

There are several ways to recognise your state of relaxation. One of these is the sensation of sounds around you seeming to be a bit further away than usual. Another is that you become aware of the weight of your body pressing down onto the floor. In no way is this last sensation unpleasant. It is only when you relax that you are aware of gravity pulling you down onto the surface on which you are lying. This becomes an extremely enjoyable feeling once you are fully relaxed.

To keep your mind pleasantly occupied, divide your attention among breathing sensations, breathing techniques, and physical techniques. If thoughts other than the ones described come into your mind, simply observe them and let them float away. Some people imagine putting these unwanted thoughts into a balloon and watching the balloon drift away. You then turn your attention back to the speaker's voice.

The 'Take-a-Break' script begins

Close your eyes. Gently point the toes and ankle of your left foot. Feel the muscles of your calf tighten, as well as the muscles of your foot. Hold that contraction for a second or so, and then let your leg relax completely. Then gently pull the toes of that foot up towards your knee to stretch the muscles you have just used. Then let your foot and lower leg relax completely.

Now turn your attention to your right leg. Gently point the toe of your right foot, moving your ankle as well. Feel the muscles of your foot tighten, and feel the muscles of your calf tighten too. Hold the tension in these muscles for a count of three; and then let your leg and foot relax completely. Next, draw the toes of your right foot up towards your right knee and feel the stretch in your calf muscles. Then let all tension go out of your lower leg and let your foot return to its most comfortable position. Feel the weight of both of your lower legs pressing your calf muscles and heels onto the floor.

Now turn your attention to your breathing. Take a breath and, as soon as your lungs are full, relax the muscles that you used to breathe in, letting the breath go right out of your body. At the next breath in, feel the sensations of the air going in through your nose, going down the back of your throat, and filling your lungs. As soon as your lungs are full, let your muscles relax completely and feel the air go out of your body of its own accord. Take in one final breath, but don't try to deepen or slow your breathing. As soon as your lungs are full again, let your body relax and let the air go out of your lungs completely. Do not force the air out. For a moment, feel the weight of your body pressing down onto the floor, and be aware that you have already started to relax.

Now turn your attention back to your legs. Starting with your right leg this time, gently tighten your right thigh, as though you were trying to straighten your leg fully. Hold that contraction for a count of two. Then let that leg relax completely. Next, turn your attention to your left leg. Tighten the front of your left leg and feel the heel of your left foot come off the ground a little. Hold that contraction for a count of two. Then let your leg relax completely. Feel the weight of both legs now pressing down onto the ground.

Turn your attention back to your breathing. This time you are going to do a breath-holding pattern. When you hold your breath in during these exercises, don't close your throat against the air in your lungs. Rather, feel the muscles of your diaphragm and ribs that you use to take in a breath and, keeping your throat open, hold the breath in using these muscles. To let the breath out, simply relax your muscles completely.

Do a three-breath cycle. Take in a breath feeling the air going in through your nose and down the back of your throat. As soon as your lungs are full (don't force this), hold the breath for a count of two. Then let the muscles relax completely, let the breath out, and feel the air flow out through your nose or mouth. As you breathe out consciously, feel how this makes your body feel even heavier, and how breathing-out is a part of relaxation. Breathe in for a second time, 'seeing' the air go in through the back of your nose, down your throat, and into your lungs. As soon as your lungs are full, hold the breath in for a count of three, and then let the breath go out of its own accord. Take in a third breath, hold for a count of three, and then let the breath go out of your body.

Take a moment to feel the weight of your body again, and to feel the beginnings of the state of deep relaxation.

Now turn your attention back to your body. From your feet through your calf muscles, the next part of your body to be in contact with the floor will be your bottom muscles. You hold a lot of tension in these muscles, so briefly tighten both buttocks, and then let your hips relax onto the floor as fully as possible. Next, feel the muscles of your lower and middle back. Are they completely relaxed? If you are not sure, move your hips and trunk around a little until you feel that your body is pressing on the floor in the most comfortable way. Take another moment to feel the weight of your body pressing on the floor—first your heels, next your calf muscles, and then your hips.

Turn your attention back to your breathing. Take in a breath, but don't hold it this time. As you breathe out, feel the air going out of your body. Once it stops going out of your body, tighten your tummy muscles very gently to get that last little bit of air out of your lungs. Hold the breath out using your tummy muscles for a count of two. Then relax your muscles and feel the air rush back into your body. Fill the lungs and feel this sensation. When your lungs are full, but without making any effort at all, stop breathing in and let the air go out again. Once the air has gone out, tighten your stomach muscles a little and get that last bit of air out. Hold the air out for a count of two. Relax completely and feel the air rush back into your lungs. Take one final breath in this sequence. Breathe in, feel the air go into your lungs, let the breath go out and, when no more air comes out, very gently tighten your tummy muscles. Hold the breath out for a count of two. Then let the breath come in. Lie there for a moment—feeling the sensation of being relaxed.

Turn your attention back to your body. The next parts of your body to contact the floor will be your middle back, your upper back, and your shoulders. To make sure that these areas are completely comfortable, gently lift your right shoulder off the floor and lower it to the floor. Then lift your left shoulder off the floor, and then lower it and let it rest on the floor. See if any part of your middle or upper back feels uncomfortable. If it does, make small gentle wriggling motions until that part of your back feels completely comfortable. Try to feel the weight of your entire body pressing onto the floor. Feel your body feeling heavier and heavier as you become more relaxed.

Now turn your attention back to your breathing. This time you are going to combine the two previous patterns. Take in a breath, feel your tummy rise under your hand and, when the breath is fully in, count to yourself—one, two, three. Immediately let your whole body relax, feel the air rush out of your body and, when no more air comes out, gently tighten your tummy muscles, breathe the last of the air out, and hold the breath out for a count of three. Immediately relax and feel the air come in through your nose and go down the back of the throat. Feel your tummy rise. Breathe in, and keep breathing in until your lungs are full. Hold the breath in for a count of three. Relax and feel the air come out of your body. Feel your tummy sink. Gently tighten your tummy muscles so that the last air comes out, and hold the breath out for a count of three. For the last cycle, again let your body relax, feel the air rush in, and hold the breath in for a count of three. Relax again, and let the air come out. Tighten your tummy muscles and hold the breath out for a count of three. Now relax completely. Savour the sensations of your body feeling completely relaxed.

Turn your attention back to your body. The last part of your body to rest on the floor is your head. Gently adjust the position of the back of your head on the floor by turning your head very slightly left or right. You might find that you need to lift your chin a little or bring your chin towards your chest a little to make the back of your neck and head feel completely comfortable on the floor. Now feel your entire body pressing onto the floor—your heels, your calf muscles, the backs of your legs, your bottom, your middle back, your upper back, your shoulders and, finally, your head. Turn your attention back to the breath now. For this cycle do absolutely nothing at all—instead concentrate fully on the sensation of five breaths in and out. Make no attempt to hold the breath in or out; make no attempt to control anything whatsoever.

[If recording this yourself, pause here for about half a minute.]

Now turn your attention to the muscles of your face. Tension is often held in different muscles in your face, so we'll run through the major muscles to make sure that you are not holding any tension in these areas.

First, clench your teeth gently. Feel the large muscles of your jaw tighten as you do. Then open your mouth as wide as you can for a second or two, and then let the muscles of your jaw relax completely and let your teeth sit in a comfortable position. You might want to move your jaw from side to side gently to make it feel comfortable. Next, gently purse your lips, pushing your mouth off your teeth. Then let your facial muscles relax completely. Then lift your eyebrows as high as you can. Feel all the muscles of your scalp that are involved in this action. Then frown. Feel how many muscles are required to do this. Then let all the tension in the muscles of your face go completely. Now visualise what you look like when seen from above. Your face is a serene mask now and completely relaxed. Your body looks soft and comfortable, and feels heavy as gravity pulls it onto the floor. This feeling of heaviness is an extremely pleasant feeling. Concentrate on it for a moment or two.

Now return your awareness to your body and your breathing at the same time. As you concentrate on your breathing, you will notice that you are breathing more slowly than usual; and yet you have made no effort to make your breathing slower. When you relax, your breathing always becomes a little slower. The weight of your body is a very pleasant sensation, and you are aware of each part of your body pressing onto the floor. You are aware that you can move your body easily, but you *choose* not to do so. Instead, you simply enjoy this sensation of deep relaxation—this state in which your body is repairing itself, and which your mind and spirit are still. Tell yourself that in ordinary daily life you will let your body relax a little each time you breathe out. Now, for the next few moments, lie on the floor enjoying this delightful sensation of deep relaxation.

[If you are recording this yourself, pause for a couple of minutes.]

Now it's time to rouse yourself from your state of relaxation. Some of the effects of this relaxation will stay with you, even when you return to normal consciousness. To come back to the normal world, press your toes away from you at the same time as you lift your arms up behind you on the floor. Press your toes away from you pulling you in one direction, and reach your arms away from you in the opposite direction. Your entire body is given a gentle stretch, and you breathe in fully, into the top of your chest as well this time. Relax your body, bring your arms back down to your sides, and repeat the actions. Point your toes, reach your arms up above and behind you, and breathe fully into your chest and abdomen. Bring your arms back to your sides and, when you are ready, roll over onto whichever side feels more comfortable. Sit up. Sit and rest for a moment or two before resuming the rest of the day.

Recommended birth positions

The following photographs show Jennifer's preferred birth positions.

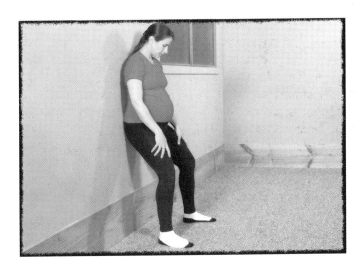

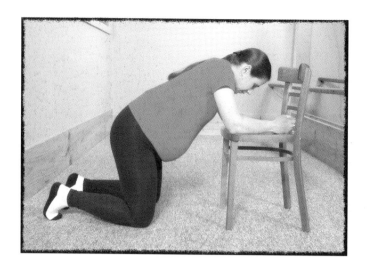

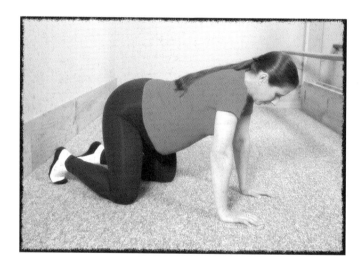

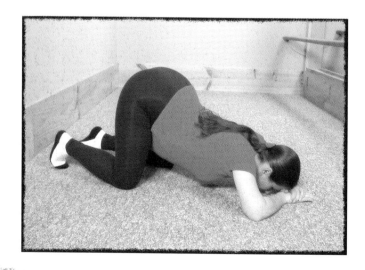

Jennifer says:

I found that moving around between these positions—a kind of pacing back and forth—was most comfortable for me during labour. You might find yourself automatically in a position that your body favours. My first labour progessed very quickly and, without thinking, I found myself on all fours (bottom photograph, opposite).

Once labour starts, your body is in control. You might feel a bit silly practising for labour now but, when the time comes, you'll be glad that you did.

If you have already practised these positions, you will be physically and psychologically comfortable moving where your body demands.

I gave birth to both Anreas and Pernille in the kneeling position.

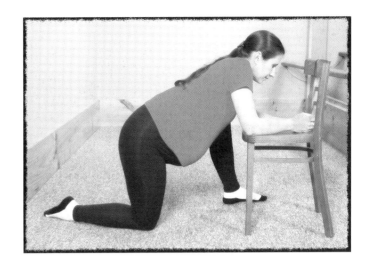

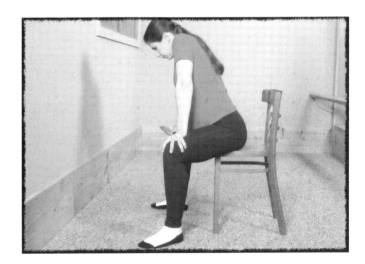

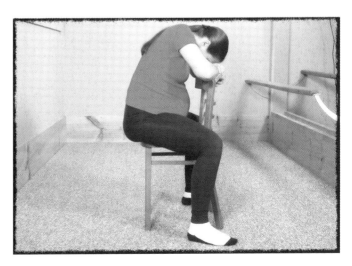

More positions overleaf

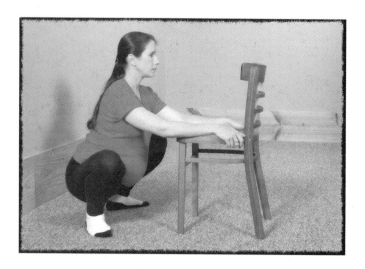

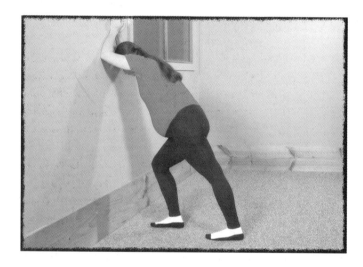

CHAPTER 3 POSTNATAL EXERCISES

Pelvic-floor and abdominal strengthening

Seven muscles, collectively called the pelvic-floor muscles, form a broad strong band between your coccyx (the tailbone at the end of the spine) and your pubic bone (at the front of the pelvis). The pelvic-floor muscles provide support for all of the internal organs. They also exert voluntary control over urination and defaecation, and provide an important element of control of your vaginal muscles.

During pregnancy, with the additional weight of the growing foetus, these muscles do increasing work. During an ordinary delivery some of these muscles are stretched very strongly. *Kegel's exercises* are most commonly used for strengthening and toning these muscles. The recommendation is to cut off the flow of urine and hold tension in the muscles used for a few seconds, before relaxing them again. Kegel's exercises are best begun as soon as you know that you are pregnant, and should be used for *relaxing* as well as *strengthening* the muscles of the pelvic floor. Following birth, these exercises will *tone* these muscles.

If you are unsure of exactly where these muscles are, try to stop the flow of urine the next time that you sit on the toilet. Feel which muscles are used to achieve this. Some experts recommend that full contraction strength is held in these muscles for a couple of seconds at a time, and that this is repeated for five to ten repetitions. Others recommend quick contracting movements followed immediately by relaxations. Use both approaches to begin your practice.

These exercises can be made more effective. If you contract the muscles that you use to stop the flow of urine, you will feel that the major effect of this action is between your perineum and your pubic bone. If you try to *increase* this contraction, you will find the muscles around your anus become increasingly involved. So, begin the contraction in the standard way and, in time, when the muscles become stronger, deepen the contraction to include all the muscles around your anus as well. In time you will be able to feel a pull from your pubic bone all the way back to your coccyx. Holding full-strength contractions will benefit you very significantly. These exercises are just as important for men as they are for women.

Start with a short contraction (a second or so), and build up the contraction—in terms of both intensity and duration. In the beginning, you might feel that there is not a great deal of strength in these muscles at all. However, in time, you will develop both control and considerable strength. The exercises can be done anywhere—on the toilet, in the shower, or even while driving a car. They can be done sitting or standing.

A few abdominal strengthening exercises are described below. Kegel's contractions can be added to any abdominal exercise to make it even more effective.

26. Lying pelvic tilt

The next strengthening exercises emphasise the abdominal muscles below your navel—in particular *transversus abdominis* (*TA*). Recent research has shown that this muscle is one of the main support systems for the lumbar spine. Following pregnancy, this muscle can become lazy or even 'switched off'. This is more likely to occur if you have had a Caesarean section.

Other research has shown that the strength relationship between the lower and upper abdominal muscles tends to favour the latter. This might increase the tendency to develop a forwards stoop.

The first photograph shows Jennifer lying on her back, with her feet comfortably on the ground with bent knees. This exercise involves a subtle movement. You will need to look at the second and third photographs closely to see the change in shape of the abdominal wall when these muscles are contracted correctly. The exercise has two parts.

Lying as shown, place your fingers inside your hip bones to feel your abdominal wall. Visualise and feel drawing your abdominal wall *directly* down towards your spine and away from your fingers. Do not tense your other abdominal muscles—a common fault is to initiate the sitting-up movement instead. Hold your abdominal wall closely into your spine for a count of three.

Now add a rearwards pelvic tilt to this general movement. Once your abdominal wall is pulled back towards the spine, use only your *abdominal* muscles to tilt the pelvis back, so that your lower back presses flat against the floor. Hold this new position for a count of three. Make sure you don't use your bottom or leg muscles to do the tilting.

Work up to ten repetitions of the pull back of your abdominal wall; then add the pelvic tilt. Work up to ten of both movements in time. Strengthening exercises need to be done only twice a week.

Once the two parts of this exercise have been mastered, you can start the exercise with Kegel's contractions. Doing this will help you to focus the effects below your navel.

Jennifer has chosen to show this exercise on the floor. However, once you become proficient it can be done sitting, or even standing. The next exercise shows the standing version of the abdominal wall pull back.

Jennifer says:

Practise, practise, practise!

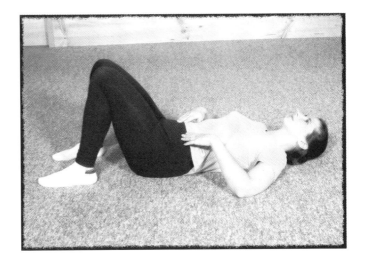

Cues

Fingers inside hip bones

Breathe in; as you breathe out, draw abdominal wall back

Hold for count of three

Tilt hips back

Lower back presses on floor

Hold for three count

Practise twice per week

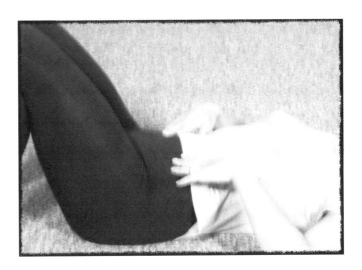

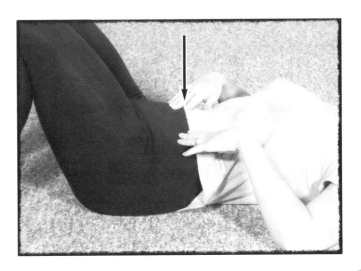

27. Standing lower abdominal pull back

The next exercise describes the first part of Exercise 26, done while in the standing position. The *corset-like* effect of toned abdominal muscles can be seen clearly.

The first photograph shows the shape of Jennifer's abdominal wall while standing with her shoulders relaxed, and her weight equally on each foot. The second photograph shows the effect of contracting only *transversus abdominis*. Her abdominal wall has been pulled back, the curve of her lumbar spine has been flattened, and her posture has become more erect. These muscles should not be contracted all the time, of course; the exercise is simply a way of waking up and strengthening these muscles.

Stand relaxed with your weight equally on each foot, and your shoulders relaxed. Using only the abdominal muscles that you used in Exercise 26, draw your abdominal wall directly back towards your spine. Hold this contraction for three to five seconds.

Make sure that, as you pull your abdominal wall back, you do not curl your trunk forwards.

If practising in front of a mirror, make sure that the shape of your lumbar spine flattens and that the shape of your middle and upper back doesn't change. Once you become proficient at holding the contractions, try breathing deeply in at out at the same time.

This exercise can be practised with your feet a few inches away from the wall and with the wall pressing against your middle back and bottom. When you perform a contraction well, you will feel your lumbar spine moving towards the wall and the whole of your spine elongating.

Do three to five repetitions of the exercise. Try the Kegel's contractions in this position too.

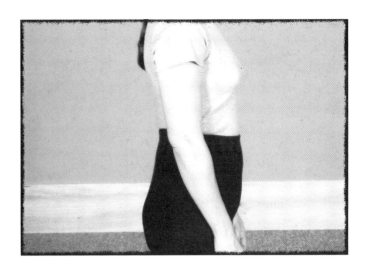

Cues

Stand relaxed

Breathe in and, as you breathe out, draw abdominal wall in

Hold for count of 3–5

Practise twice per week

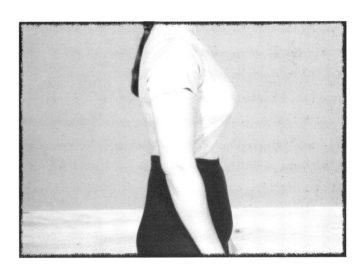

28. Lying 'crunches' (general abdominal)

Many of you will be familiar with this exercise in some form or another. You can see it being done badly in any gym, anywhere in the world! The most important aspect of form is the speed—the exercise must be done slowly.

Jennifer is demonstrating a number of different arm positions—from the easiest to the most difficult. Start with the easiest ones first, work your way up to ten repetitions at this level and, when you feel confident, use the more difficult arm positions, twice per week.

Jennifer is resting her legs on the back of a chair. This is not essential. The exercise can be done with the same leg position that we used in Exercise 26. However, using the chair allows your legs to relax completely and helps you learn how to do the exercise properly.

Lie on the floor with your legs on a chair as shown, and with your arms outstretched alongside you.

Breathe in. As you breathe out, draw your lower abdominal wall towards your spine—as in the previous exercises. While breathing out a small amount, slowly lift your head off the floor. Once your head is off the floor and your chin moves towards your chest, tighten your stomach muscles so that your body is curled. *To avoid straining your neck, make sure that your head does not lag behind your shoulders.* Most people feel the effects of this exercise in their front neck muscles. Some tightness in that area is evidence that the muscles are being worked and is no cause for alarm.

You might find that pressing the centre of your tongue to the roof of your mouth helps to activate your deep neck muscles—and this makes lifting your head easier.

The second photograph shows the fully contracted position. Hold this for a count of two. Slowly relax and let yourself move back to the floor, breathing in as you do so. Relax on the floor for an instant, and repeat.

Once you become proficient at the movement, the Kegel exercises can be added. Perform the Kegel contractions, draw your abdominal wall to the spine, and add the curling movement.

The more difficult version is the same in all respects except that your arms are folded on your chest.

The hardest version of the exercise is to place your fingers on your forehead or at your temples. All other directions remain the same. It is better not to lift your head with your hands. If your neck tires first (quite common with beginners) this is an indication that these muscles also need strengthening. In a short time, the main effects will be felt in the abdominal muscles.

Jennifer says:

Start with the easiest hand position. Work up to ten repetitions. When you can do ten, try the more difficult hand positions.

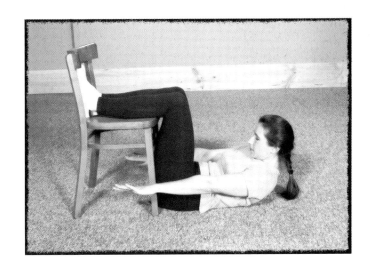

Cues

Do exercise *slowly!*

Arms by sides

Curl chin to chest

Slowly curl shoulders

Hold for 'one, two'

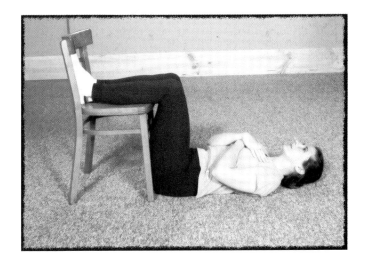

More difficult:

Arms across chest

Most difficult:

Fingers at temples

Practise twice per week

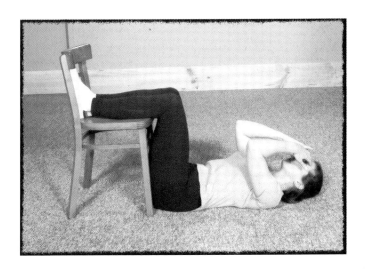

29. Lying bent leg rotations

This is the most difficult of the abdominal exercises in terms of strength required to do the movement properly. *All* trunk muscles are involved in this movement—the muscles at the front of the abdominal wall, the muscles at the sides, and the superficial and deep back muscles. It is a complete trunk-strengthening exercise. The easiest form of the exercise is quite a gentle movement, and the most intense form of the exercise is very difficult. You can choose any grade of intensity between these two extremes.

No matter how strong you are, start with the easiest version of the exercise. Look at the first and third photographs in the sequence. Notice that Jennifer's lumbar spine is perfectly straight in the rotated position. This is achieved by her aiming her knees towards the outstretched arm. This form direction is essential to avoid hyperextending (bending backwards) at the lumbar spine, and is necessary to avoid discomfort in that area.

Stretch your arms out to the side as shown (palm up or palm down), and press your arms into the floor to hold your trunk stable. Lift your knees off the floor and fold your legs. You can cross your ankles if you wish. While thinking about aiming your knees towards your hands, take in a breath, pull your abdominal wall back towards your spine and lower your knees to the floor. *Do not let your legs rest on the floor.*

As soon as your outer thigh touches the floor, begin the lifting action. Make sure that all your *trunk* muscles are involved in the exercise. This is achieved by concentrating on the muscles below your navel and around the outside of your waist.

Use the easiest version of the exercise until you can do eight repetitions to each side. When you feel ready, you can make the exercise more difficult by slightly straightening your legs.

If you become very strong, you can do the exercise with fully straight legs. Do not be in a hurry to do this advanced version.

As with all abdominal exercises, make sure the exercise is done *slowly*. As a guide, it should take you three to five seconds to lift your legs off the floor. Try to keep tension in all of your abdominal muscles as you do the movement. Count to yourself: 'one-thousand, two-thousand, three-thousand . . . '.

Jennifer says:

This will work all your trunk muscles, including those of your waist and lower back. All your strengthening exercises should be done in the one session. It will take only five minutes.

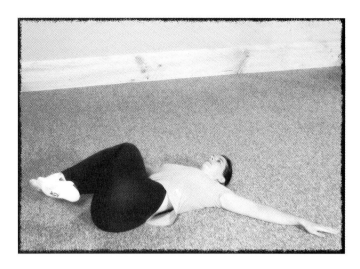

Cues

Easiest:

Bend knees

Arms out to sides

Breathe in

Pull lower abdominals in

Slowly lower legs

Aim knees at hand

Use whole waist to lift

Perform movements slowly

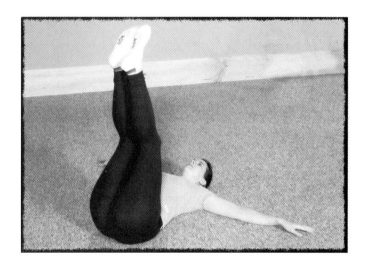

More difficult:

Half straighten legs

Most difficult:

Straight legs

Practise twice per week

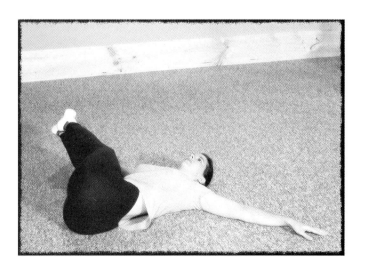

Additional and stronger stretches

Now that your baby has been born, there will be much lifting to do around the house. In particular, the middle-back and upper-back muscles will be doing more work than usual. The next exercise provides a very pleasing stretch for the middle of your back, and its effects are concentrated between your shoulder blades.

30. Middle and upper back

This can be done from the floor, from a bench, or from the front of a chair. Sit as shown and hold your knees. Let your body slump. Tighten your abdominal muscles and push your hips backwards. Hold this stretch position for a few breaths.

To make the sensation stronger, pull your shoulders towards your knees while maintaining the trunk position.

To move the main focus of the stretch, hold *one* knee with both hands. Pull yourself gently towards this knee, while maintaining the rolled-back hips and slumped-back position. The stretch will be felt under the opposite shoulder.

Contractions can increase the effect. Go back to the first version of the exercise. Holding yourself in a stretch position with your arms, pull back gently with your *trunk* muscles. The *restretch* is applied by using your arms to pull yourself a little closer to your knees, while maintaining the rolled-back hips and slumped-back position. The contraction can also be applied to the single-knee version of the exercise.

Both versions of the exercise can be done sitting on your feet, or sitting cross-legged.

Hold the final positions for a few breaths. Stand up and loosely swing your arms around you to relax the muscles completely.

Jennifer says:

Great for the upper back. It's simple, it's easy, and it works. One of my favourites!

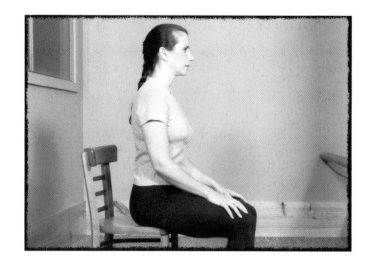

Cues

Sit and hold knees

Let body slump

Tighten abdominals

Pull on arms to stretch

One knee to move stretch

C–R:
Can use both knees or one

Pull back with trunk

Use arms to increase stretch

Breathe!

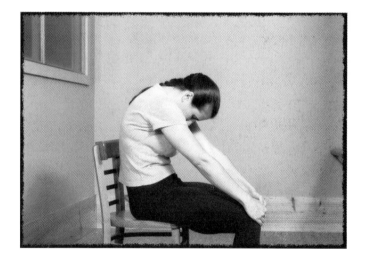

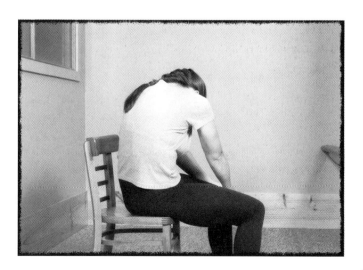

31. Hip flexors

Sacroiliac joint pain is not uncommon following childbirth. During childbirth, the *sacrum* and the *ilia* (the large bones that make up the bulk of your pelvis) move significantly in relation to each other, to allow your baby's head to pass through. One source of joint pain might be an incomplete return of these bones to their previous positions.

Lower-back pain postpartum can be due to many factors—reduced tension in your abdominal muscles, lingering tightness in your lower-back muscles, residual tension in your hip flexors, or a combination of these factors. All of these can contribute to an exaggerated anterior pelvic tilt. One of the possible causes has been addressed with the abdominal-strengthening exercises outlined above. The present exercise (Exercise 31) is offered to address another dimension of the problem. Loosening these muscles can also help to ease sacroiliac joint pain.

The first photograph shows the general form. The exercise is designed to move your leg behind your body while keeping your spine in the neutral position. Jennifer has moved into a gentle stretch position, and has kept her hips square (at 90 degrees to the line made by her legs) and her trunk erect. She has added the posterior pelvic tilt that we have practised. Using her bottom muscles she has strongly 'tucked her tail under' and this has reduced the curve in her lumbar spine. A stretch sensation will be felt at the front of her hip, at the top of her leg.

The second photograph shows her moving both hips *forwards* from this position, while keeping her tail tucked under. This provides a strong stretch for all the muscles that lift her knee towards her chest.

A *contraction* can be effective in creating new movement at your hip joint in this position. Gently *try* to drag your back knee forwards. It will not move, because friction holds it on the floor. Hold the contraction for a count of five.

Take in a breath and relax your back leg. Tuck your tail under again, and *restretch* by moving both hips further forwards in the stretch direction. Hold your final position for at least five breaths in and out. The contraction and restretch sequence can be repeated.

The final photographs shows Jennifer stretching with her back leg *next* to the support. This might be more stable (one hand is holding her front knee; the other on the support). See which works best for you. Exercise 31 is an extremely strong stretch, and needs to be done properly *twice a week only*.

Jennifer says:

Make a special effort to include this in your routine.

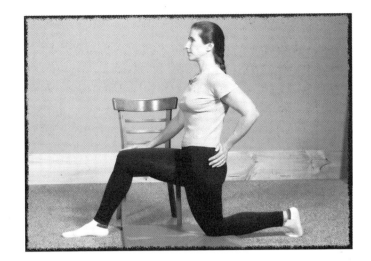

Cues

Square hips to line of legs

Trunk vertical

Back straight

Tuck tail under

Move into stretch

C–R:

Pull back knee forwards

Restretch: go further into stretch

Hold final position for five breaths

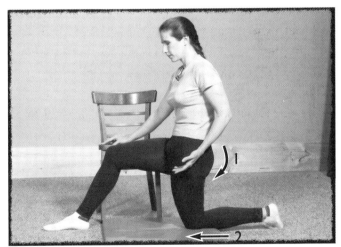

Tail tuck (1) and contraction direction (2)

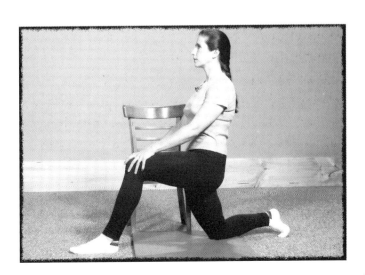

25. Floor legs apart (revisited)

Exercise 11 (Floor relaxed lunge) addressed the *causes* of some kinds of lower-back pain. The present exercise revisited (Exercise 25, Floor legs apart) addresses the *effects*. Most people feel the discomfort and tension of lower-back pain in the superficial and deep muscles of the lumbar spine, between the spine and the hips. A stronger version of Exercise 25 is now presented.

The first photograph shows the alignment of the starting position. Your spine is inside the line of the leg that you are stretching over, and your arm is reached out and off your body as far as you can. This stretches most of the muscles in your back and trunk.

The second photograph shows a more intense version, where your top arm is holding on to a strap around your foot. This allows you to apply a little more tension in the sideways direction, and adds the large muscles under your shoulder to the stretch. Ensure that you breathe fully—your lower ribs on the side you are bending away from will move as you do, helping the stretch.

The final photograph shows the most intense position, in which Jennifer's bottom shoulder is placed *inside* the line of her leg. Her top shoulder is rolled back outside her leg, and her top arm is holding firmly onto her foot. Her bottom hand is holding the shin of her folded leg—which helps the rotation aspect of this excellent exercise.

Recall that once you have achieved a stretch in the sideways direction, you can move the focus from the outside of your waist further around into your lumbar spine by rolling your top shoulder forwards in small increments.

Contractions can loosen tight muscles in this exercise. Assuming that you are holding on to the strap around your foot or holding on to the foot itself, once you are in the stretch position use the muscles that are being stretched to try to pull your hand gently away from your support for a count of five.

To *restretch*, move your body further in the initial stretch direction. As you roll your shoulder further forwards to move the stretch, *contractions* can be done at any point where you feel there might be a benefit. Make sure you breathe deeply during the whole of the stretch.

Make sure you stretch the other side. Finish your stretch session with a forwards-bending or a rotation movement that makes your whole body feel comfortable.

Jennifer says:

Do what you can. Don't overstretch.

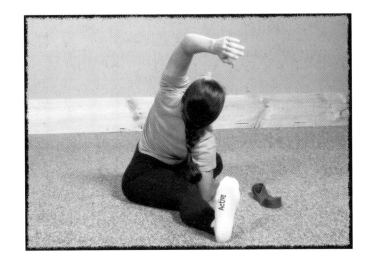

Cues

Incline trunk to side

Hold foot or strap

Extend arm out above body

Breathe deeply

Roll shoulder forwards
to move stretch

Use arms to recover

C–R:
While holding, pull back

Restretch: go further
in stretch direction

Breathe!

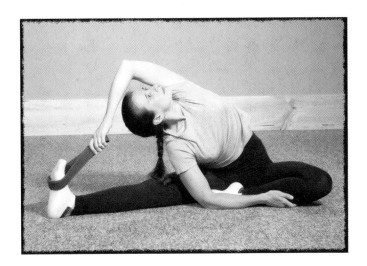

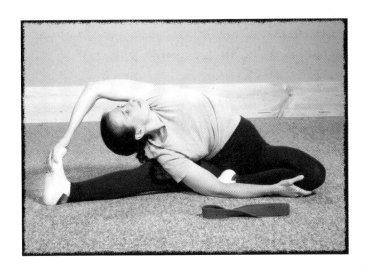

32. Legs apart forwards bend

Exercise 25 is a perfect warm-up for Exercise 32, the final stretching exercise in this book. In its completed form it is one of the major poses from dance, yoga, and gymnastics (in which it is a compulsory aspect of the floor routine). The exercise stretches all the muscles at the back of, and inside, the legs. There are two parts.

In the first photograph, Jennifer is bending over her straight leg, with her back straight. Doing this will stretch the hamstrings of the leg you are bending over. If you cannot reach this far forwards without bending your back, loop a strap around your foot.

Concentrate on holding your back as straight as possible. If you wish to loosen your hamstrings with a *contraction*, once you are in a good stretch position lift your chest up to straighten your back further. Then pull back on your hands (or strap) gently—using the muscles at the back of your leg. After taking in a breath, use your arms to pull you a little closer to your leg to *restretch*.

The second photograph shows the final part of this exercise. With a perfectly straight back, Jennifer has leant forwards from her hips. This action stretches the muscles on the insides of both legs in addition to the muscles at the back of her legs. If you feel the stretch sensation in your lower back, you are letting it bend! Sit up, restraighten your back, and lean forwards again.

If you are tight, sit on a cushion. This will tip you forwards slightly and make the stretch position easier to hold. If you have a stable support in front of you, hold it and use it to straighten your back. Then pull yourself further forwards.

If you have something to hold (you might be able to hold your feet, or a support) a *contraction* can improve your position. Making sure your back is straight, lift your chest and very gently pull back, using the muscles at the back of your leg. (You can also use the muscles on the inside of your leg if you are far enough forwards.) A longer contraction (ten to fifteen seconds) will be effective.

Apply the *restretch* by pulling yourself slowly and gently further forwards. Hold the final position for five to ten breaths. Finish your workout with any stretch that you find relaxes your body.

The last photograph shows a perfect final position—a goal to reach one day!

Jennifer says:

Not an essential stretch, but pursue if you like a challenge.

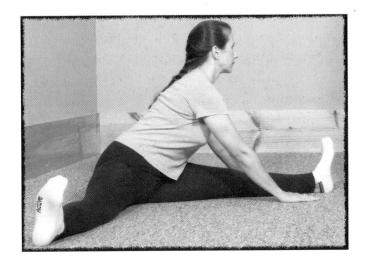

Cues

Hold trunk straight

Incline from the hips

C–R:
While holding, pull back

Restretch: go further
in stretch direction

Breathe!

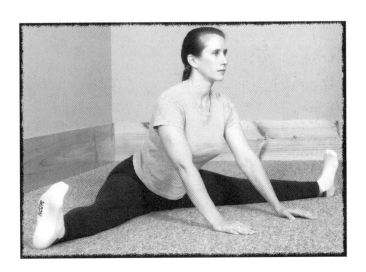

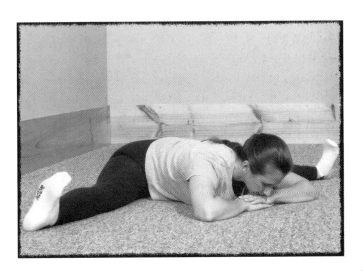

Chapter 4 Sensible Eating

Some basic concepts

It is helpful to begin with some terms commonly used in discussing nutrition. This will be of assistance in understanding the recommendations contained in the rest of the chapter.

The components of food can be classified into three broad categories of *macronutrients*. These are *protein*, *fat*, and *carbohydrate*. All contain *micronutrients*. These are *vitamins* and *minerals*.

The energy content of food is now measured in kilojoules. Energy content used to be measured in kilocalories—commonly called, simply, Calories (with a capital C). One Calorie equals approximately 4.2 kilojoules.

Protein

Protein (from the Greek *proteios*, meaning 'primary'), is made up of *amino acids*. There are nine *essential amino acids* (eleven for premature babies).

The proteins made up of these amino acids are the basic elements of:
- more than 50 000 *enzymes* (essential to all chemical reactions in our bodies);
- blood plasma; and
- the structural proteins (for example, collagen, part of connective tissue, and muscle proteins).

Foods supplying proteins include:
- meat, eggs, fish, and dairy products (these are high in proteins);
- legumes, such as beans and lentils (moderately high);
- whole grains (medium);
- vegetables and fruit (low, but still significant).

Women require about 50 grams of protein daily. Pregnant women need an extra 30 grams per day (80 grams in total), and lactating mothers require about 20 grams extra per day (70 grams per day). Men require approximately 75 grams daily. These intakes of protein must include the essential amino acids in proportions suitable for our bodies.

Protein contains approximately 16.8 kilojoules (4 Calories) of energy per gram.

Fat

Fat is comprised of *fatty acids*. Some fats are said to be *saturated* (for example, animal fats) and others are are said to be *unsaturated* (for example, olive oil). These terms refer to their chemical structure.

Just as there are *essential* amino acids, there are also *essential fatty acids* (EFAs) that our bodies must have daily. These are used to make all other required fatty acids. Fats make up (in part):
- hormones;
- cell membranes;
- nerve sheaths; and
- cellular transport mechanisms.

They are therefore essential to life.

Our bodies are made mostly of protein and fat, with some minerals.

Because fat contains 37.8 kilojoules (9 Calories) per gram, it is a concentrated source of energy.

Carbohydrate

Carbohydrate is the preferred energy source for our bodies. All vegetables, fruit, and grains are sources of carbohydrate. They are usually classified as being *simple carbohydrates* (sugars) and *complex carbohydrates* (starches).

Gylcaemic index (*GI*) is useful measure of carbohydrate activity in the body. This indicates how rapidly a food is converted to glucose and how quickly blood glucose, the body's fuel, rises.

Carbohydrate, like protein, contains about 16.8 kilojoules (4 Calories) of energy per gram.

Micronutrients

The micronutrients are:
- *vitamins* (the absence of which leads to specific disease); and
- *minerals* (which are essential for chemical and metabolic processes).

Some vitamins are *antioxidants*. This means that they bond with *free radicals*—which are byproducts of oxygen reactions in the body, and harmful in excess. This bonding leads to elimination of the antioxidants from our bodies.

Taking a new look at food

The majority of articles on food tend to concentrate on the kilojoule (or Calorie) content of food. Because fats contain the most kilojoules, these articles therefore tend to concentrate on the fat content of food. This has serious limitations for pregnant and lactating women. It is better to think about food in terms of the combinations of foods that will provide optimal *nutrition* for you and your child.

Expectant women (indeed, any person interested in health!) should try to minimise or avoid less desirable foods and maximise desirable foods in their diet. Desirable foods maximise nutrition and thus provide kilojoules that are beneficial. Less desirable foods have *high kilojoule density* and *low nutritional density*. The term 'nutritional density' refers to the extent to which the fifty nutrients that are essential to life are found in a particular type of food.

Let us look at a few examples.

White bread is very dense in kilojoules. One slice of white bread has roughly the same number of kilojoules as more than three and a half cups of broccoli—but the broccoli contains a huge range of additional vitamins, minerals, and phytonutrients (see page 137 for more on phytonutrients).

White sugar is rich in carbohydrate, but contains no other nutrients—in fact, its digestion *removes* various micronutrients from the body, and its kilojoule density is relatively high. In contrast, spinach is rich in a large variety of nutrients. However, because of its vegetable structure, it is low in kilojoules.

As far as possible, you should try to eat food that is relatively *kilojoule sparse* and relatively *nutrition rich* because this ensures that the amount of nutrition you get in each mouthful of food is optimised. In the process, you will be avoiding unwanted weight gain (body fat). The total amount of energy that you need will depend on your activity level.

Another way of understanding this is to say that if you eat more of your food from the list of 'What to include' (page 124), you can eat a greater amount of food to achieve your desired kilojoule total, and each mouthful is giving you more in terms of nutrition.

And remember that all foods eaten in excess of energy requirements are stored as fat.

When choosing food, it is helpful to know that some complex carbohydrates have a very high glycaemic index (GI). In general, lower GI foods are preferable to higher GI foods because foods with a lower GI provide energy over a longer period. Pure glucose is given the highest rating of 100 and is the benchmark against which other carbohydrates are measured. The basic GI of a food can be altered significantly by *refinement.* For example, a boiled new potato has a GI of 62, whereas instant potato from a packet has a GI of 83. Whole grains have low GIs (for example, crushed wheat used in Lebanese food is less than 50), but refined grain products (bread and biscuits) can be 90 or more. Although many grain products are described as 'complex carbohydrates', they can behave like a simple sugar once digested, so consideration of GI can be helpful.

Notice that many refined foods are found in the list of 'What to minimise or exclude' (page 124). The refining process generally increases carbohydrate density (the amount of carbohydrate in any volume of food). The refining processes also usually remove essential fatty acids and other highly reactive food substances. The result is a tendency to lower nutrient density. These substances are removed in refining to increase the food's shelf life.

Therefore, if you are concerned with maximising nutrition, you should eat more unrefined food sources. Of course, some foods are nutritionally *and* relatively kilojoule dense (for example, meat).

Desirable foods

These lists are only a rough guide. They are designed to help you look at food a different way, and to assist you to choose food that is better for you.

High-quality protein and low-to-medium saturated fat
- lean meat (beef, lamb, pork, venison, game meats)
- chicken (remove skin)
- fish (especially salmon, tuna); fresh, smoked, or canned

Medium-quality protein and medium-density carbohydrates
- dried beans
- kidney beans
- lentils
- chick-peas
- cracked wheat
- brown rice
- soy beans (canned beans are OK)
- tofu

Medium-quality protein and beneficial fat; high nutrition
- brazil nuts
- pecan nuts
- almonds
- cashews
- hazel nuts
- avocado

Low-density carbohydrates; high nutrition (fruit with medium-to-high GI)
- grapes (black grapes best; but also green grapes)
- bananas
- oranges and other citrus fruits
- apples and pears
- figs (fresh)
- dates (fresh)
- cherries

Low-density carbohydrates; high nutrition (vegetables with relatively low GI)
- capsicum
- spinach
- broccoli
- cauliflower
- potatoes (boiled)
- celery
- zucchini
- Chinese vegetables
- onion
- garlic
- ginger
- peas
- beans
- carrots (raw)
- Brussels sprouts
- other sprouts (mung, soy, alfalfa)

Medium-high density carbohydrate; low-medium protein; good nutrition
- 'heavy' breads (dark rye, pumpernickel)
- slow-cooking oats
- whole-grain pasta
- skim milk
- skim-milk yoghurt

Less desirable foods

Medium-high GI carbohydrate; low protein; kilojoule-dense
- breakfast cereals (packaged)
- rice (white)
- bread (white; 'light')
- pasta
- potatoes (instant)
- rice (instant)
- fruit juices
- sugar (raw)
- honey
- potato chips
- biscuits
- cakes
- instant noodles
- soups (packaged)
- chocolate
- fruit (canned; versions with no added sugar better)

High saturated fat; trans-fatty acids; low-medium protein; kilojoule-dense
- 'TV' dinners (including 'low-fat')
- pizza
- hamburgers
- 'fast' or 'junk' food

Medium-low density carbohydrate; low protein; high GI
- carrots (cooked)
- potatoes (baked or fried)
- parsnips (cooked)
- broad beans
- dried apricots
- baked beans (canned)

Foods with no known nutritional value
- cordials
- sweet carbonated drinks
- white (refined) sugar
- sugar-coated food

Some suggestions for meals of the day

In the pages that follow is a list of what foods to include in a sensible eating plan (and what to minimise or avoid), followed by a discussion of the reasons for our recommendations.

What to include

Breakfast
- grain-based source (unrefined if possible);
- protein source, or health shake (recipe suggestions below);
- piece of fresh fruit.

Mid-morning snack
- piece of fruit plus piece of cheese; or
- closed handful of raw mixed nuts and piece of fruit; or
- two to three tablespoons of cottage cheese and fruit; or
- small tin of tuna or salmon and piece of fruit; or
- meal replacement (drink or bar).

Lunch
- palm-sized lean protein source;
- two-hand-sized salad; or
- hand-sized lightly cooked vegetables; or
- half-and-half salad and cooked vegetables (approximately two-hand-sized);
- piece of fruit (optional).

Afternoon snack
- same as mid-morning snack.

Dinner
- protein source;
- fresh vegetables (starchy and leafy);
- piece of fruit.

What to minimise or exclude
- recreational drugs;
- coffee and tea;
- refined packaged food sources;
- 'fast' food;
- fried food;
- foods that are kilojoule-rich and nutrient-sparse (high GI foods);
- excessive kilojoules;
- foods rich in saturated fats;
- sweet carbonated drinks and refined sugar;
- low-fat packaged foods; and
- 'convenience' food.

Reasons for recommendations

Breakfast

In our list of 'What to include' (page 124), the following recommendations were made for breakfast:

- grain-based source (unrefined if possible);
- protein source, or health shake (recipe suggestions below);
- piece of fresh fruit.

Some thoughts on each of these is included below.

Grain-based source

There are two traditional Australian breakfasts—which might be termed the 'bacon-and-eggs approach' and the 'cereal (grain) approach'. Both have good aspects, and not-so-good aspects. (Cereals are considered immediately below; for bacon and eggs see under 'Protein source', below.)

The best grains for breakfast are ordinary oats. Not only are they a source of *slow-release energy* (low GI of around 40), but also they contain gamma linolenic acid. Indeed, oats are one of the very few plant sources of this desirable fatty acid. You can add some honey, fruit, and milk (dairy or soy) if you wish. Note that the more 'instant' forms of oats generally have a higher GI.

Less-desirable sources of carbohydrate are the more-refined breakfast cereals. Try to get organically sourced and wholegrain cereals if you can. The least desirable grain-based carbohydrate sources are the even more refined versions of these foods, and the worst ones have the individual flakes covered in sugar.

Other desirable sources of unrefined carbohydrates are the heavier (in weight) of the wholegrain breads, pumpernickel (dark rye) bread, and mixed-grain breads. Less desirable are the ordinary brown breads, and the least desirable is white bread—even if the label does say that it is fortified with extra fibre. If you are eating sensibly, fibre will not be a problem.

Protein source

There are many sources of protein.

If you eat animal protein, a couple of soft-boiled or poached eggs, or an omelette made of two or three eggs (with your favourite filling) is an excellent choice. If you are concerned about excess cholesterol intake, simply do not eat some of the yolks. (The yolk contains some cholesterol, but many nutritious substances too.) If you have two or three soft-boiled eggs for breakfast, you can choose to have the yolk of one and eat only the whites of the other two. (However, it is always a good idea to have at least one yolk.)

Bacon and eggs supply a good amount of protein—often missing in many modern breakfasts—but can supply significant amounts of saturated fat. Reserve for special occasions, and use lean bacon!

Other good protein sources are cheese and yoghurt (especially good with mixed raw nuts, fresh fruit, and/or honey for additional flavour).

Health shake

A health shake is a good way to 'jump-start' your morning with excellent quality nutrition.

The basic liquid into which the other ingredients is blended is a matter of choice. You can use 50:50 fruit juice and water, or you can use a low-fat high-calcium milk source (or a soy-milk equivalent). If you prefer, you can use whole milk. However, if you are adding yoghurt and other products to it, the end mixture can be quite thick and heavy.

To the basic liquid, add two or three generous tablespoons of yoghurt (flavoured or non-flavoured). The organic ones are best, or you can make your own. If you look at the contents of many of the brands of yoghurt that you find on the supermarket shelves, you will be amazed at how much sugar they contain. The best of the organic yoghurts are flavoured with real fruit and do not contain preservatives or any other extra chemicals. A raw egg or two can be added.

Add some fresh fruit. Bananas taste good, and they blend extremely well, but any ripe fruit can be used. Some people don't like the idea of mixing citrus fruit with a milk-based drink (if you are using milk or similar as the base), but the resulting mixture has an excellent taste.

If you feel that you need additional protein at the beginning of the day, you can add about 10 grams (about a tablespoon or two) of a suitable protein powder. Whey protein powder is said to have the highest 'biological value'. This means that more of the protein in the powder is taken up by the body than a similar amount of another protein source, but really any powdered protein will do. If you are on a budget, use two or three tablespoons of skim milk powder. Skim milk contains *casein* which is an excellent high-quality protein. Vegetarians can fortify their shakes with soy protein, available from a health food shop. If you need extra fibre, Psyllium husks (one or two teaspoons) can add the right kind of fibre—good insurance with no 'down' side, in any case.

The final part of the health shake is a tablespoon of an oil containing the essential fatty acids (EFAs). These are linolenic acid (LNA) and linoleic acid (LA). Research suggests that the average Western diet is low in LNA. The addition of oil to the basic mixture makes the resulting shake taste creamy and delicious, even if you haven't used yoghurt. Flax seed oil is the best source of LNA, and is obtainable from a health food shop. It is stored in dark bottles and must be kept in the refrigerator.

This is a useful place to discuss the fats that everyone is afraid of. *Cholesterol*, a saturated fat, is an essential substance in the body, but does not need to be eaten. Cholesterol is produced by the liver and is a major fraction of brain tissue and the nerves of the body. High blood cholesterol is usually a result of genetics, but good dietary habits (increasing EFAs and fibre) and adopting the relaxation strategies described in Chapter 2 can be beneficial. *Trans-fatty acids* are toxins produced by heating and refining oils, and using oils to fry. In the pursuit of good health, these cooking practices need to be minimised. Sufficient EFAs and antioxidants (such as vitamins A, C, and E) should be included in your diet to help your body process trans-fatty acids.

LNA is also found in soy bean and walnut oils, and dark green leafy vegetables. The other essential fatty acid, LA, is found in safflower, sunflower, soy bean, sesame, and flax seed oil. Buy oils that contain EFAs from a health food shop, and choose cold-pressed organic sources. These oils *cannot* be used for cooking.

A note for lactating mothers: the Nursing Mothers Association of Australia (NMAA) states that 'if you are eating enough for your own energy requirements, the fatty acid pattern in your milk will resemble that of your diet' (Carafellam 1996, see References, page 146). This is good reason for asking yourself if you have sufficient EFAs in your diet.

The breakfast is finished with an optional piece of fresh fruit (discussed below).

Mid-morning snack

In our list of 'What to include' (page 124), the following recommendations were made for mid-morning snack:

- piece of fruit plus piece of cheese; or
- closed handful of raw mixed nuts and piece of fruit; or
- two to three tablespoons of cottage cheese and fruit; or
- small tin of tuna or salmon and piece of fruit; or
- meal replacement (drink or bar).

Some thoughts on each of these are included below.

Piece of fruit plus piece of cheese

Any ripe fresh fruit is a good source of simple (and some complex) carbohydrates, minerals, vitamins, and fibre. Ripe bananas are especially good. The notion of complex carbohydrates can be a bit misleading however, because the bonds between the glucose molecules (that give rise to the term 'complex') are easily broken down. This process begins in your mouth (during chewing) and is normally completed in your stomach (during the first stage of digestion). Some complex carbohydrate sources can raise your blood sugar level quite quickly. However, because you are having only one piece of fruit and a small amount of protein together, this will not be a problem. Any cheese will do, but if you are concerned about your intake of cholesterol, consider a low-fat variety.

Closed handful of raw mixed nuts and piece of fruit

All nut varieties contain beneficial fatty acids. If the nuts are roasted, the chemical composition of some of the fatty acids can be changed, so it is probably best to eat nuts raw. Eating mixed raw nuts ensures that a greater variety of essential fatty acids is consumed. Nuts are also a good source of protein, contain no cholesterol, and have minimal amounts of saturated fats.

Two to three tablespoons of cottage (or ricotta) cheese and fruit

Cottage cheese is made from milk and contains casein, an excellent high-quality protein. It is also low in saturated fat. Add this to a piece of fresh fruit and you have an excellent snack.

Small tin of tuna/salmon and piece of fruit

Fish is a form of protein that cans very well. Two fatty acids found in the oils of cold-water fish are part of the same omega 3 fatty acid family that includes LNA. Salmon is a migratory fish, and it has a high oil content.

The oil found in fish is good for your body. Recent research suggests that increasing your consumption of these fatty acids can help prevent cardiovascular disease. The extent to which these fatty acids are changed by the canning process is unclear. A better source of these oils is sliced smoked salmon (found in supermarkets).

Together with a piece of fruit, you obtain a small amount of excellent-quality protein and a small amount of easily digested carbohydrate.

Meal replacement (drink or bar; check label for the 'extras')

There is an increasing variety of meal-replacement bars or powders on the market. Careful reading of the labels reveals an extraordinary variation in the proportions of carbohydrate, protein, and fat in these products. If you want to use a meal replacement, choose one in which these various nutrients are present in approximately equal amounts in terms of kilojoules. Many manufactured substances can be used to make the final product taste and feel like food. Check the labels!

Be aware that if you use low-fat or fat-free meal replacements, the rate at which the carbohydrate enters your bloodstream is faster than it would be if some fat is present in the product, and this can raise the blood sugar level of some people a bit too rapidly. For this reason, the bars that have some fat in them (depending on the kind of fat) are generally preferable to the ones with little or no fat.

Lunch

In our list of 'What to include' (page 124), the following recommendations were made for lunch:
- palm-sized lean protein source;
- two-hand-sized salad; or
- hand-sized lightly cooked vegetables; or
- half-and-half salad and cooked vegetables (approximately two-hand-sized);
- piece of fruit (optional).

Some thoughts on each of these are included below.

Palm-sized lean protein source

The basis of our sensible eating plan is to maximise the amount of nutrition in the food that we eat and minimise the number of 'empty' kilojoules (little or no nutrition). A quick way of assessing your diet is to consider it in terms of how much carbohydrate, protein, and fat are likely to be in it.

The various *Zone* books by Barry Sears, and *Body of Life* by Bill Phillips, both recommend an 'eyeballing' method for assessing protein and carbohydrate quantities. This is because the body can assimilate only about 25 grams of protein at any one sitting. The rest is excreted or stored. Accordingly, it is a good idea to have just the right amount of any nutrient. A palm-sized piece of lean protein will contain 25–40 grams of protein, depending on its thickness (and the size of your palm!). To help you assess,

100 grams of steak contains about 25 grams of protein. Vegetarians (vegans or lacto-ovo vegetarians) will need to give some thought as to how much protein (and what proportion of which amino acids) is being consumed in their favourite food sources.

Two-hand-sized salad

Have some raw vegetables at most main meals, before or during the rest of the meal. Raw vegetables contain many enzymes that the body can use to help digest proteins, carbohydrates, and fats in the food that you eat. To ensure the greatest variety of phytonutrients, try to have as many *colours* in the salad as you can.

Many vegetables can be added to salads. These include varieties of lettuce (common in many salads), beetroot and carrot (can be grated), beans and peas (added raw), and broccoli and other brassicas (lightly steamed before adding). There are, of course, many other vegetables that can be added.

Nuts can be added to salads to increase the protein and (beneficial) fat content.

If you use one of the recommended oils as part of your dressing, salads provide a very convenient way of getting some of the two essential fatty acids.

Eat roughly 'hand-sized' if you are having other vegetables; increase the salad serving size if not.

Because these foods are low in carbohydrate density, you can eat as much as you like.

Hand-sized lightly cooked vegetables

The recommendation of a 'palm-sized' piece of lean protein (above) provides a simple assessment of how much protein to eat at each meal. This also applies to the suggestion to have a *hand*-sized serving of lightly cooked vegetables. This amount provides a good balance to the palm-sized protein source that you are combining with this meal. Together, you will get an excellent source of carbohydrates, proteins, and fats.

In addition, the vegetables (raw or lightly cooked) will provide you with many of the vitamins and minerals that are needed in daily life. Your body requires nutrition 'as needed'. This means that you need to have all of the fifty essential nutrients (discussed below) almost every day. This means, for example, that is not good to have a big serving of spinach on Monday, and not eat any other dark-green leafy vegetables until Friday.

Food is cooked to make it more palatable, and some nutrients are released by the process. However, many enzymes are denatured or destroyed if food is cooked for too long or too hot. This is why we recommend *lightly* cooked vegetables.

The best way to cook vegetables is to use a non-stick pan, or to cook in a quarter of a teaspoon of butter or coconut oil. Add a quarter of a cup of water, fit a tight lid, and steam the vegetables. Add some of your favourite oil as a dressing after cooking. Recommended oils include virgin olive (Australia is making some wonderful olive oils now) or a mixture of the oils that will supply the essential fatty acids.

Half-and-half salad and cooked vegetables (approx. two-hand-sized)

An even better suggestion to increase enzyme and nutrient intake in the diet is to have a salad and some cooked vegetables which, together, form roughly a hand-sized serving. This is fiddly, however, and you might choose to have your cooked vegetables at lunch and your salad at dinner, or vice versa. Have a slice of a heavy bread, if you wish.

Piece of fruit (optional)

To finish lunch, you can have a piece of fruit. But this is optional, and you might simply be too full to eat another thing! If you do leave fruit out of your lunch, you can have it for an afternoon snack.

Afternoon snack

Same as for mid-morning snack.

Dinner

In our list of 'What to include' (page 124), the following recommendations were made for lunch:

- protein source;
- fresh vegetables (starchy and leafy);
- piece of fruit.

Some thoughts on each of these are included below.

Protein source

We need a protein source at dinner too. We have suggested using the palm of your hand as a rough assessment of the desired 25–30 grams of protein. But where does that leave someone who wants to eat spaghetti bolognese or similar for dinner? The answer is that the same 'palm-sized' vs 'hand-sized' proportion as a guide still applies, but consider a small kitchen ladle to be equivalent to a palm-sized serving. Assuming a sauce that contains protein and carbohydrate, consider the ladle volume to be the protein part, and have an equivalent amount of the pasta. Compared with vegetables, pasta is carbohydrate *dense*, so a smaller amount is required for balance. Have some additional low GI vegetables on the side.

A salad with many different kinds of vegetables is an excellent complement to this meal. However, starchy vegetables are *denser* carbohydrate sources and, if you choose a lean palm-sized protein source, you will probably want to include some of these starchy vegetables as well—to make sure that you are getting sufficient carbohydrates. (You might also have a slice of one of the heavy breads.) Starchy vegetables include the tubers (including potato, sweet potato, and pumpkin).

Avoid deep-frying these vegetables. Deep-frying in otherwise good vegetable oil changes the oil and creates substances called trans-fatty acids, which are no good for your body at all. It is far better to steam or boil the vegetables and add some sort of good oil at the serving stage.

If you wish, have a tasty ripe piece of fruit to finish the meal.

Reasons for minimising or excluding

Recreational drugs

This might seem obvious as a suggestion for a pregnant woman, but it is nevertheless worth emphasising. Once you know you are pregnant it is very wise to avoid all recreational drugs—including alcohol. The most important reason is that in developed countries, folate deficiency is often linked to excessive consumption of alcohol. Alcohol limits the absorption of this vitamin. Inadequate folate is definitely associated with neural tube abnormalities in the foetus (producing disorders such as spina bifida) and might well be associated with miscarriage. A list of foods containing folate can be found on page 139.

Another reason for our strong recommendation against the use of recreational drugs during pregnancy is the increased likelihood of various other birth defects. Apart from alcohol, recreational drugs include tobacco, stimulants of various kinds, marijuana, and other non-prescription drugs.

You should also check all *prescription* drugs with your doctor to make sure that these drugs pose no threat to the developing foetus.

Tea and coffee

Green teas, in particular, have been found to be good sources of various antioxidants. This is good news if you like tea! However, tea is a mild *diuretic* (that is, it causes the body to lose water), so make sure that you have your tea reasonably weak and have a glass of water for every cup.

Coffee, unfortunately, doesn't seem to have any benefits according to many researchers—unless you count its great taste! If you consume too many cups (usually reckoned at more than three per day) you will encounter one of the disadvantages of this drink—too much caffeine. This can make you irritable and can make your hands tremble. Coffee, depending on the strength, is a stronger diuretic than tea, so have a glass of water with every cup you drink to offset this effect.

Anecdotal evidence suggests that coffee can affect the foetus. Many women note increased foetal activity if they drink coffee.

Expectant women are advised to limit both tea and coffee.

Refined packaged food sources

These are not recommended because of the refinement process which removes some, and sometimes many, of the original nutrients.

The exception is packaged frozen vegetables. Unlike supermarket produce, it is picked and 'snap frozen' when ripe. Research suggests that some of the desirable phytonutrients form during the ripening period. With fruit, this is in the last few days of ripening. Canned fruit can be used when fresh fruit is not available. Use the 'no added sugar' varieties.

Because ripening is so important, organic fruit and vegetables are desirable. They are picked closer to this ideal time before being brought to market.

'Fast' foods

'Fast foods' include takeaway hamburgers, pizzas, and the like. The carbohydrates of these foods are usually kilojoule-dense and nutrition-poor, and a high proportion of the fats are saturated.

In addition, the method of manufacture of these foods tends to produce trans-fatty acids. Trans-fatty acids are broken down much more slowly in your body than the recommended fatty acids, producing much larger amounts of free radicals. Some researchers have linked high amounts of trans-fatty acids to an increased susceptibility to various cardiovascular and degenerative diseases.

Fast foods also usually contain a large (often surprisingly large) amount of sugar and salt.

Margarine vs butter

Trans-fatty acids, in addition to being found in fried foods, are also found in hydrogenated vegetable oil products, in many packaged foods (check the label to be sure), and in margarine. All margarines start their life as vegetable oils—some of which are unsaturated and some of which are polyunsaturated. All are liquid at room temperature.

During manufacturing, these oils are *hydrogenated* (an artificial saturation process) to make them more or less solid at room temperature, and thus able to imitate the spreadability and texture of butter. This process leaves the final product full of trans-fatty acids (which, as explained above, should be minimised).

Products that are a combination of butter and margarine must be treated with caution for the same reasons.

Butter might be better, after all.

Fried food

The inadvisability of eating deep-fried food has been mentioned above, but how can you cook all of the other food that you eat?

One way is to use a variation on a traditional Chinese method of stir-frying. Instead of throwing oil into the bottom of the wok or a non-stick frying pan—and heating vigorously until it smokes, as some recipe books suggest—put in a ladleful of water or stock, instead of the oil. Depending on the recipe, you can substitute canned or fresh tomatoes. To this, add garlic and the other seasonings. Once the seasonings and other condiments have been cooked sufficiently, add the vegetables and other ingredients. Immediately cover the pan or wok with a tight-fitting lid.

Cooking this way ensures that the minimum amount of nutrients will be lost and that the food will be steamed and partially boiled. This method will ensure that the cooking temperature of the foods will not go above 100 degrees Celsius—the highest temperature that cooking water can reach.

Keeping the cooking temperature at or below 100 degrees Celsius reduces the conversion of fatty acids to trans-fatty acids. In addition, because the temperature is relatively low, some of the enzymes and other volatile food elements remain largely unchanged.

When you remove the lid and are ready to serve, you can add a good-quality oil. Olive oils and other oils can be added in this way, and the taste is different from cooking with oils. It is, in fact, delicious.

As well as the other benefits, the oil itself hasn't been changed by the cooking process. Therefore, the benefits of the particular oil that you add will be experienced.

Most foods that are traditionally fried can be cooked in this way. Of course, you can't make chips like this! However, chips and other fried (or roasted) vegetables should not be part of your usual diet. Keep these for special occasions!

Foods that are kilojoule-rich and nutrient-sparse (high GI foods)

The ratio of kilojoules (or Calories) to nutrients, and the GI, of any food can be changed by its method of preparation. For example, carrot juice has a much higher GI than a whole raw carrot, and is missing most of the beneficial fibre contained in a whole raw carrot. To take another example, whole grains are excellent sources of all sorts of vitamins, minerals, fibre, essential fatty acids, proteins, and carbohydrate. However, the refining process used to produce the final form of the food that most of us eat removes almost all of the nutritional components except the carbohydrate.

As mentioned previously, although white bread is often described as a good source of complex carbohydrate, it can have a GI as high as 90. Surprisingly, ordinary white table sugar has a GI of only 65, which suggests that its rate of conversion to glucose is significantly slower than white bread. (For a quick comparison, according to Brand Miller et al. 1996, cherries have a GI of only 22, apples 36, and bananas approximately 55.)

The biggest surprise in looking at GIs is that many 'complex' carbohydrates are treated like simple sugars by your body. Foods in the 'desirable' list above have lower GIs on average, and foods in the 'less-desirable' list have higher GIs. (Some foods in the 'desirable' list have relatively high GIs, but these are nutritionally dense as well.)

Don't cut out all of the things that you really love to eat. Rather, use the lists to think about whether or not the food you are about to eat is located more at one end of the nutrition spectrum than the other, and make adjustments to suit. During pregnancy, the food that you eat feeds both you and your baby. Every nutrient advantage that you can manage is to the benefit of both of you.

Sweet carbonated drinks and refined sugar

These drinks are a perfect example of a kilojoule-dense nutrient-sparse food. The amount of refined sugar contained in sweet popular beverages is extraordinary. For example, a standard can of drink can contain 10–20 teaspoons of refined sugar. If you consume one or two cans (or bottles) of these drinks a day, you are getting a huge number of extra kilojoules that are of no nutritional benefit.

Minimise these products as far as possible. Much the same goes for the commercially made fruit juices. These also contain lots of sugar and not too many nutrients. You are much better eating a piece of fruit instead.

Some years ago, a book came onto the market with the alarming title *Pure, White and Deadly*. The book referred to ordinary refined white table sugar (sucrose). It now seems likely that the alleged dangers of white table sugar were exaggerated, but it is a good idea to minimise the amount of additional sugar added in cooking—simply because sugar is pure carbohydrate with no other nutrients. There might be some benefit in using unrefined sugar (rather than the refined version), but any nutritional benefits are likely to be small.

So what should you do about desserts? Desserts (like chips) are best reserved for special occasions. This is because desserts are usually relatively kilojoule-dense compared with the rest of the meal. Of course, you can calculate the approximate number of kilojoules (Calories) that you want to eat in a meal, and make the necessary adjustments. But if you are eating for two people, there are grounds for reducing the consumption of desserts and increasing the consumption of more nutritious foods.

There are, however, some desserts that are nutritious in their own right. These sorts of desserts can simply be considered as part of the total meal.

Low-fat packaged sources

Labels advertising 'low cholesterol' can be found on all manner of foods these days—including avocados in supermarkets and greengrocers' shops. This preoccupation with 'cholesterol' is reflected in the stated goals of a US Senate Select Committee on Nutrition and Human Needs which published its report in 1977 (Grills and Bosscher 1981). These goals focus on the prevention of diet-related diseases such as obesity, cardiovascular diseases, diabetes, and dental disease. Among the goals was a recommendation to reduce overall fat consumption from approximately 40% to about 30% of energy intake (not a huge reduction) and a further recommendation to reduce cholesterol consumption to about 300 milligrams per day. Most people have absolutely no idea of what 300 milligrams a day of cholesterol means. (I certainly don't!)

Much has been made of the association of cholesterol and other saturated fats with cardiovascular disease, and this is one of the reasons for fat-free and low-fat foods being promoted so aggressively. The problem with this recommendation is that it makes no distinction between beneficial and harmful fats. A further problem with very low-fat products is that the remainder of their composition is largely carbohydrate. On page 121, we noted that if complex carbohydrate is eaten without the GI-lowering effects of the right kind of fat and fibre, the conversion of complex carbohydrate to glucose can be very rapid.

Another associated problem is that in the effort to make the processed food as low in fat as possible while retaining the 'taste' of fats, the use of various substances not found in the original food has increased. For example, commercially prepared yoghurt contains all sorts of chemicals that are not in the original milk (soy, dairy, or goat's milk) that is used to make traditional yoghurt. Minimising the intake of these additional substances is probably prudent.

Artificial sweeteners should also be regarded with caution. Sears (1999, page 281) states that aspartame 'should never have become part of the food supply'. Use natural sweeteners sensibly.

'Convenience' foods

Many of the remarks made about other foods also apply to convenience foods. The only real 'convenience' here is preparation time. If one is eating with nutrition in mind, the 'convenience' might turn out to be an illusion.

The basis of the sensible eating plan

The following section provides more detail on certain elements of nutrition. You might feel that you already have enough information on which to base your eating plan. However, if you feel that more detail will assist your food choices, read on!

Fifty nutrients are essential to support human life. They are discussed below.

Essential amino acids

There are twenty-two amino acids, but only nine (or eleven for premature infants) are 'essential' in your diet. If your body has the full spectrum of these essential amino acids your body can make the remainder.

All animal sources of protein are 'complete'—meaning that all the essential amino acids are present in a ratio that is favourable for humans. However, all animal protein sources contain saturated fat as well.

Vegetarian sources vary in the favourability of their ratios. For example, corn has been traditionally eaten with beans in some parts of the world. Corn on its own lacks an amino acid called lycine, but beans have this amino acid in abundance. Together, corn and beans contain all the essential amino acids in a favourable ratio.

Recent research suggests that your body has an amino acid 'pool'—which exists for half a day to a number of days. If you are a vegetarian and you eat a protein source that is low in a particular amino acid, you probably don't have to worry too much. At the next meal you will probably eat a food containing the missing amino acid. However, if you wish to be meticulous, and you think that there is a benefit from eating complete proteins at *every* meal, give some thought to combining your proteins.

Another traditional protein combination is rice and sesame seeds. There are several other similar combinations. *Diet for a Small Planet* (see References, page 147), an excellent source of nutritional advice, is an invaluable source of this kind of information. Note that all the grain sources have some high-quality protein, and this content is higher if the grain source is unrefined (unprocessed).

Essential fatty acids

There are only two essential fatty acids. If you have the two *essential* fatty acids in your diet in the right proportion, your body can make all of the other fatty acids needed for health.

The opinions of researchers differ considerably on the ideal proportion of omega 3 to omega 6 fatty acids. Erasmus (*Fats that Heal, Fats that Kill*, see References page 146) suggests that most people in the modern Western world are significantly deficient in LNA, an omega 3 fatty acid. If your diet in the past has been high in saturated fats and you have eaten a lot of fried foods (and hence have had significant amounts of trans-fatty acids in your body), Erasmus recommends adding extra omega 3 fatty acids to your daily intake for six months or so.

The best vegetable source of this particular fatty acid is the oil derived from flax seeds. This is available in the refrigerated section of health food shops. This is a particularly reactive substance, and for this reason it is sold in opaque containers, and must be kept refrigerated. Never use this for cooking. It is best added to foods after cooking, or on top of other breakfast cereals or yoghurt. A tablespoon or two is the recommended daily amount. Once you feel that you have achieved some sort of balance in the fatty acids in your body, you might wish to change the proportion of the two essential fatty acids.

Apparently hemp oil contains a more or less ideal balance for human consumption—but I haven't seen any hemp oil available in my local health food shop! A better way is to combine flax-seed oil with one of the other cold-pressed vegetable oils that is rich in omega 6 fatty acids. These include safflower oil, sunflower oil, and sesame-seed oil. Again, do not use these oils for cooking—they are damaged by heat. They should be mixed up and used as a salad dressing, or used as a topping on other foods.

The main fatty acid of olive oil is oleic acid. This is not an essential fatty acid, but it might have benefits for people at risk of cardiovascular disease—*provided* it is virgin or extra virgin olive oil. These terms refer to the pressing process that removes the oil from the olives, and virgin or extra virgin olive oil are produced in a way that maintains the maximum nutritive value of the oil. The term 'light' (and other terms that you see on oil labels) tells you that it is *not* virgin—and hence processed in some way. Such oils should be minimised or avoided.

Minerals

In Australia, until recently, vitamin and mineral preparations were not permitted to contain selenium—even though Australian soils are said to be the poorest in selenium of any soils in the world. The reason for this prohibition was that, like many substances, selenium is toxic in large doses. However, selenium is now a permitted mineral in supplements.

The results of a full blood assay can be very helpful in planning food choices and possible mineral supplementation. This test is available on Medicare if recommended by a doctor, so you might wish to discuss this with your medical practitioner.

Of particular interest to expectant women are three minerals—iron, calcium, and magnesium.

Anaemia (low haemoglobin level) is caused by insufficient available iron. Sometimes women can feel tired and be told that their haemoglobin levels are 'within normal limits'. Despite this apparent 'normality', many women find that iron supplements can help, and can increase their energy significantly. A daily supplement of one tablet per day (each containing about 100 milligrams of elemental iron) is recommended. These are available 'over the counter' at pharmacies.

You might prefer to address this problem through diet rather than supplements. Constipation can be a side-effect of iron tablets, *if* there is insufficient fibre in your diet. Everyone Jennifer talked to about this problem, including midwives, believes constipation is a problem regardless of dietary fibre intake. Consider a couple of teaspoons of Psyllium husks with all meals if this is the case for you. Dark-green leafy vegetables are an excellent source of dietary iron.

Calcium and magnesium are required for healthy bones—both in yourself and your baby. The recommended daily allowance of calcium is 800–1200 milligrams per day, and the recommended allowance for magnesium is 300–400 milligrams per day. Some recent US research suggests that magnesium is also an important mineral in avoiding or reducing the likelihood of cardiovascular problems. To be on the safe side, it is probably a good idea to have a daily mineral and vitamin supplement obtained from some reputable source. (Floridix is a preparation that Jennifer used.)

The best supplements contain different forms of the various minerals, some of these being described as 'chelated'. This means that the element is coated, or prepared with a particular amino acid, so that the substance in question can be better assimilated by your body. If you are concerned about any possible effects that such a supplement might have, discuss it with your doctor.

Vitamins

There are thirteen recognised vitamins. No new vitamins have been named since 1954, even though thousands of phytonutrients (compounds contained in plants) have been discovered since then. The term 'vitamin', and how it can be applied to particular substances, is subject to two strict criteria. The first is that the absence of the substance in the diet must be causally linked to a particular disease. The second is that the addition of that substance to the diet must be able to reverse the course of the disease. For example, the absence of vitamin C causes scurvy, and the reintroduction of the vitamin reverses the disease process.

However, these criteria have proven to be too restrictive in terms of adding to the list of vitamins. Some researchers feel that many phytonutrients (not classed as vitamins) have important health-giving properties—even if they are not essential. Certain phytonutrients are likely to be extremely important in helping your body deal with cancer cells that are produced every day. For example, the brassica family (including cauliflower, Brussels sprouts, and broccoli) is said to contain a number of phytonutrients that are beneficial in halting the course of some cancers. This is another good reason to get a significant fraction of your day's carbohydrates from a variety of vegetables—because they each contain different phytonutrients in various proportions.

Some of the vitamins are called 'antioxidants'. These include vitamins A, C, and E. If you are going to supplement vitamin A intake, it is better to take beta-carotene (a double molecule of vitamin A that your body breaks down as needed), or to make sure that you eat as many different coloured vegetables as possible. The antioxidants combine with substances called 'free radicals'—which are produced in all oxidative reactions in the body (such as those required to metabolise trans-fatty acids). Some researchers claim that excess free radicals in your body can damage your chromosomes, and hence compromise your body's ability to reproduce its cells accurately. This might be a significant part of the ageing process. Most of the cells in your body are renewed within a brief two-year period—that is, at the end of a two-period you are actually composed of different molecules. In this sense, 'we are what we eat'—because our bodies can be 'remade' only from the things that we take in each day.

Among the B group of vitamins is folic acid (vitamin B_9). This vitamin is essential to the developing foetus. On page 139, you will find a chart reproduced from a recent source showing which ordinary foods contain folate, and in what amounts.

The recommended daily allowance of cobalmin (vitamin B_{12}) is extremely small (0.006 milligram per day). However, it is a crucial nutrient, and vegetarians should know that strict vegans are likely to have low B_{12} stores. If you suspect that you might be low in vitamin B_{12}, it is worth getting a vitamin and mineral supplement that has adequate amounts of this vitamin.

Vitamin D is manufactured by the body and its manufacture is accelerated by exposure to ordinary sunlight.

Be aware of the interaction between vitamins and minerals on the one hand, and the macronutrients (protein, carbohydrate, and fat) on the other. As mentioned, *all* the minerals and vitamins are necessary for the effective metabolism of the macronutrients.

Foods containing folate

Folate helps to prevent neural tube (spinal cord) abnormalities in the foetus. These abnormalities include spina bifida. Folate might also be important in preventing miscarriage in the early stages of pregnancy.

The recommended daily allowance (RDA) for folate is 400 micrograms. This should be taken by all women who might become pregnant because it is important to have adequate folate at the very beginning of pregnancy (indeed, before women know that they are pregnant), as well as during confirmed pregnancy. Women who have a history of giving birth to babies with neural tube disorders should take as much as 4 *milligrams* per day.

Adequate folate must therefore be consumed, and most women should probably take supplements in addition to being aware of the following dietary sources. If you have any queries about this important matter, consult your medical practitioner.

Folate and food sources

Food	Serving size	Amount (mg)	Daily value (%) *
Chicken liver	115 gm (3.5 oz)	770	193
Breakfast cereals	0.5 to 1.5 cup	100 to 400	25 to 100
Braised beef liver	115 gm (3.5 oz)	217	54
Lentils (cooked)	0.5 cup	180	45
Chick-peas	0.5 cup	141	35
Asparagus	0.5 cup	132	33
Spinach (cooked)	0.5 cup	131	33
Black beans	0.5 cup	128	32
Burrito with beans	2	118	30
Kidney beans	0.5 cup	115	29
Baked beans & pork	1 cup	92	23
Lima beans	0.5 cup	78	20
Tomato juice	1 cup	48	12
Brussels sprouts	0.5 cup	47	12
Orange	1 medium	47	12
Broccoli (cooked)	0.5 cup	39	10
French fries	large order	38	10
Wheat germ	2 tbsp	38	10
Fortified white bread	1 slice	38	10

* Daily value refers to percentage of folate RDA. That is, this is the percentage of the suggested daily requirement that you will get from the various sources listed.

Source: *Food Values of Portions Commonly Used*, <www.parenthoodweb.com>

Energy sources

There are no essential carbohydrates in the way that there are essential amino acids and essential fatty acids. However, everyone needs good sources of energy.

The best sources of carbohydrates are wholegrain products, fruits, and vegetables. Commonly, food pyramids separate these foods, giving the impression that the carbohydrates that they contain are somehow fundamentally different—but they are not. Most of the food pyramids have grain sources at the bottom, and recommend that they should form the major fraction of your carbohydrate intake. If the food from these grain sources is largely unrefined, this is good advice. Such food is full of minerals, vitamins, good-quality protein, beneficial fatty acids, and carbohydrate. However, in the refining process, much of the good nutrients are lost and you are left with relatively nutrient-poor carbohydrate.

All vegetables and fruits are excellent sources of carbohydrate and are comparatively rich in nutrients. It is therefore advisable to use these for your carbohydrates—rather than emphasising the grain-based sources.

Another consideration is the glycaemic index of a food source. In one sense, the concept of a glycaemic index is deceptive. For example, if you combine a high GI food with a low GI one (depending on the precise nature of the foods involved), the glycaemic index of the whole meal will be a figure between the index of each food. It is desirable to get a balance of high and low glycaemic foods in the same meal, to avoid excessive increases in blood sugar following eating.

A further dimension to consider in assessing energy sources is the amount and kind of fat and fibre present in the same meal. Both of these decrease the overall glycaemic index of the meal.

Finally, individual reactions to particular foods will vary the GIs by very significant amounts. A variation of 20% or more can be seen in the figures cited (see Brand Miller et al. 1996, pages 207–40).

Oxygen

This element is an obvious necessity. No one can survive more than a few minutes without oxygen. Make sure that you have enough fresh air blowing through your house during the day. If you work in an office, it is essential to get out of the office environment at some time—perhaps at lunchtime—and expose yourself to cleaner air (it is to be hoped that it is cleaner!) than you find inside a typical office. Walking at any time of the day that you can manage it is good too.

Light

The action of light on the skin helps your body create the essential vitamin D. The action of light on the retina also stimulates the pineal gland and helps some people to avoid the unpleasantness of seasonal mood disorder—sometimes called 'seasonal affective disorder' (SAD).

Water

Recommendations for how much water one should consume daily vary quite widely. It depends on your body weight, level of activity, and so on. However, a minimum recommendation for water consumption is two litres per day.

If you are concerned about your water intake, substitute a glass of water for the cup of coffee or cup of tea that you might otherwise have.

Because water forms approximately 70% of your body weight, it is wise to give some thought to the purity of the water you drink. Benchtop water purifiers can be helpful, or drink best-quality bottled water. Read the label on bottled water to determine the source—the information might surprise you. Tap water in Australia is usually safe to drink. Another way to increase your fluid intake is to have nutritious soups at mealtimes. If you like fruit juices, but are concerned about getting too many kilojoules, dilute the juice by half with water.

Movement

In a book concerned with stretching and strengthening exercises, the recommendation for movement might seem superfluous. However, it is an essential consideration on a daily basis and, when taken together with the need for oxygen and light, provides a good reason for getting out of the house or out of the office at least once a day, and going for a walk.

Every authority considers walking to be excellent exercise—provided that walking doesn't give you neck or back pain, or aggravate some pre-existing condition. If this is the case, swimming can be substituted for walking. Going for a walk gives you a chance to open your lungs fully, to breathe deeply, and to make sure that you get enough direct sunlight (to stimulate your brain and help your body make vitamin D).

Walking is also fun! Of course, if the conditions are too hot or too bright, make sure that you go out with a hat on and cover your skin. The last thing you want is a case of sunburn while pursuing your health goals.

Breastfeeding

Breastfeeding is desirable. Apart from the health benefits—the full extent of which have become obvious only in the last ten years or so—women tend to return to their previous weight much more quickly if they breastfeed. One reason for this might simply be the huge energy requirement of lactation.

Maureen Minchin (*Breastfeeding Matters*, see References, page 147) identified what she called the 'six o'clock starvation syndrome'. This can be attributed to the energy cost of lactation. Breastfeeding mothers should eat as many nutritious snacks as you feel you need. The reasons for this are obvious—not only do you need to run around and do the normal things that people do in their daily lives, but also you need to have enough energy to produce sufficient milk for your new baby. When you are breastfeeding, you will need to give additional regard to what you eat. In Jennifer's case, for example, eating chick-peas had an undesirable effect on her daughter immediately following breastfeeding.

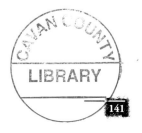

PUTTING IT ALL TOGETHER

Although this book is primarily concerned with stretching and strengthening exercises, the relaxation exercises of Chapter 2 and the nutritional advice of Chapter 4 are arguably the most important recommendations to follow on a daily basis, given today's stressful lifestyles. Use the information in the book the following way.

Exercises

Prenatal

If you are prenatal, start practising the exercises of Chapter 1 as soon as convenient. Follow the recommendations of Chapter 2, especially the one about doing relaxation practice instead of the exercises if you feel tired! In any case, do the stretching exercises at most three times a week. If you already practise some form of exercise involving stretching (yoga, for example), you can divide your practice and do something six days a week. But do *different* exercises on successive days, and do as many relaxation practices as your schedule allows (but no less than three times a week).

For example, you might do rotation and hip-flexor or front-thigh exercises on one day, and do legs-apart and hamstring exercises on the next. In this way your body will have time to adapt to the new stresses and your improvements will be faster. If you are following a routine of doing stretches three times per week, do your relaxation practice on the alternate days, and have one day off. If you swim or run, do your stretching exercises following these activities. Any time you feel tired, do a relaxation practice instead. You will be glad that you did.

Postnatal

If you are postnatal, start the pelvic-floor exercises immediately and start the strengthening exercises as soon as you can. Any of the prenatal stretching exercises can also be done.

Nutrition

The nutritional information can be used three times a day, or more if you snack. Food contains the most important chemicals we put into our bodies, and every meal is important. 'We are what we eat', so begin improving your nutrition today. If you want additional information on this complex subject, read the recommended books and go on from there.

You are on a fascinating journey, involving many great changes. Slow down, relax (and breathe!), and enjoy the experience.

ACKNOWLEDGMENTS

Being neither an expectant woman nor a nursing mother, I relied heavily on my collaborator, Jennifer Cristaudo. Unfailingly good natured—even when asked to retake a particular exercise on our video shoot for the fourth or fifth time—Jennifer remained almost supernaturally patient. These are the characteristics that typify her approach to teaching beginning students—making her the ideal person with whom to collaborate on a book of this nature. Jennifer also has a great sense of humour, which makes the somewhat arduous process of making a teaching video and taking endless photographs of the same exercise a much easier task that it otherwise might have been. Jennifer has also annotated a number of the references, and added her views on most of the exercises.

Jennifer's partner, Chris Bishop, was also helpful—especially with an extended discussion we had about food. Chapter 4 (on sensible eating) proved to be the most difficult chapter to write, even with the resources of the best-qualified and most erudite of the current crop of writers on this vexed subject. Dr Greg Laughlin made some very helpful suggestions about organising the material in this chapter and read quite a few drafts, and the chapter benefited greatly thereby. In trying to write a practical guide about such a huge topic, the challenge was in deciding what *not* to include. Apart from the sheer scope of the subject, the current best-selling books on diet present wildly varying recommendations on dietary proportions of protein, fat, and carbohydrate— and *all* claim to be backed up by impeccable science!

Susan Read, another member of the *P&F* team and whose special interest is nutrition, contributed in a number of wide-ranging conversations. My close friend Bill Giles, a medical ecologist, also made significant contributions. Bill's special interest is the consideration of food as medicine, finding substance to support the ancient oriental wisdom that 'food is medicine or poison, depending on the receiving body'. I believe that this will be a growth area in nutrition.

With regard to the strengthening exercises, I thank my friend Paul Chek for demonstrating the importance of *transversus abdominis* to me (and effective ways of cuing its activation), and for reaffirming my belief that the trunk muscles are the most important muscles in the body (and the most forgotten, too!).

Because I wished to avoid typing another book, early in the planning I decided to dictate instead. Like magic, the text appeared in email, typed up by the ever-helpful Morag <typepool@ozemail.com.au>. This allowed for a more conversational approach, and for a far more relaxed working environment. (I am trying to take the advice that I always give to my patients!) It also helped me to avoid the 'overuse' problems that are always a possibility for poor typists.

The graphic artist with whom I work, Jeremy Mears, has moved to another country location. This time any 'typos' are the responsibility of Reggie, his cockatiel (rather than the cats, as on previous books)! Not only did Jeremy do all of the laying-up and design of the book, and manipulate all the photographs, but also he operated the video camera that we used to make the accompanying videotape. As I have mentioned elsewhere, Jeremy is a wonderful person to work with and never loses his temper! As those of you who have written a book will know, it is anything but a relaxing business and, in the same period of time that the latest book was written, Jeremy and I also completely rebuilt our website. Log on to it sometime at <www.posture-and-flexibility.com.au>, and let us know what you think of it (and the book and video, too). We incorporate all feedback on all the projects we are involved with, and we are *really* interested in knowing what you think.

This is the place to acknowledge publicly the support and contributions of the whole *P&F* teaching team, especially the senior teachers (Olivia Allnutt, Jennifer Cristaudo, and Dr Greg Laughlin) and our national organiser, the indefatigable and indispensable Sharon Clark. As mentioned elsewhere, the *P&F* system is a vibrant (too vibrant, sometimes) self-determining body now—one which continually surprises and delights me. And because the organisation has moved out of Canberra to involve other parts of Australia, its diversity continues to expand—to the benefit of us all. To think that this was something that I started just to make sure I did some stretching each week is amazing! Wholehearted thanks to you all.

Sincere gratitude is expressed to the editor of this book, the witty, intelligent, erudite (and fantastically precise!) Dr Ross Gilham. His influence is everywhere in the book, particularly the organisation of the Preface, Introduction, and the chapter on sensible eating. His influence is also seen in the physical layout and styling of the book—Jeremy and I learnt a great deal. Ross tidied up many of my discursive remarks which, because, I dictated the text, were even more numerous than usual! The process of writing, editing, discussing, further editing, getting the corrections into the original MS (and relaying the text, as its length and organisation changed) and proofreading (with *its* corrections) all required a steady hand on the wheel—and Ross has been that steady hand. Any errors of fact remain mine, of course.

Thank you, too, to the senior staff of Simon & Schuster, Julie Stanton and Brigitta Doyle. We have had many interesting conversations and when one is thinking about the next book in the most general way *before* ideas are set, the importance of these conversations cannot be underestimated. And I have also appreciated David Rodrick's advice on many subjects over the years.

Others in my immediate environment have made invaluable contributions to my life (that aspect of existence that tries to continue while writing!). You know who you are, and I thank you sincerely. It is a commonplace for authors to observe, but true nonetheless, that without your help the book could not have been written.

KIT LAUGHLIN
MARCH 2001
CANBERRA

REFERENCES AND READING LIST

Balaskas, J., 1991, *New Active Birth*, Thorsons, London.

Jennifer comments:

A 'must-have' modern classic. If you read only one other book about pregnancy it has to be this one. Essential reading for birth partners also.

Brand Miller, J., Foster-Powell, K., & Colaguiri, S., 1996, *Glycaemic Index Factor*, Hodder & Stoughton, Sydney.

Kit comments:

A moderately useful guide to the glycaemic indexes (GIs) of common foods. The large variations in individual response to the different foods tested might surprise you—plus or minus ten or fifteen points is not unusual. Many of the foods reported are Canadian.

Carafellam J. (ed.), 1996, *Breastfeeding . . . naturally*, Nursing Mothers Association of Australia (NMAA), Sydney.

Jennifer comments:

Everything you need to know about breastfeeding from Australia's largest self-help group. Practical, straightforward advice concerning every aspect of breastfeeding. The NMAA has groups in most centres and provides free counselling assistance 24 hours a day. Don't hesitate to contact the NMAA at: PO Box 4000, Glen Iris, Victoria 3146; telephone: 03 9885 085; email: <nursingm@nmaa.asn.au>; website: <www.nmaa.asn.au>.

Erasmus, U., 1993 (5th printing, 1997), *Fats that heal, Fats that kill*, Alive Books, Burnaby, Canada.

Kit comments:

The best reference on the complex chemistry of the world of lipids will be found in these pages, along with a wealth of practical advice on sensible nutrition. Erasmus also contextualises the processes used by the food-manufacturing industries in terms of science, technology, and politics.

Grills, N. J. & Bosscher, M. V., 1981, *Manual of Nutrition and Diet Therapy*, Macmillan Publishing Co., New York.

Kit comments:

This manual contains excellent recommendations for people with special dietary needs. Comparing the values given in this reference with the latest figures presented on the worldwide web by the United States and Australian governments reveals that very little has changed in recommended dietary allowances (RDAs) in the past twenty years.

Kitzinger, S., 1988, *Freedom and Choice in Childbirth*, Penguin, London.

Jennifer comments:

Unfortunately no longer in print, but you might be able to pick up a secondhand copy or find it in your local library. Excellent discussion of the many issues of pregnancy and birthing options.

Kitzinger, S., 1997, *The New Pregnancy and Childbirth*, Doubleday/Dorling, London.

Jennifer comments:
A fully updated version of the 1980 classic by one of the foremost writers on women's health.

Lappé, F. M., 1971 (revised edn 1982), *Diet for a Small Planet*, Random House, New York.

Kit comments:
This was the first best-selling book on food to locate Western dietary practices in a context of fossil fuel, land, water, fertiliser budgets, and the activities of food-producing and food-manufacturing industries globally. Contains hundreds of recipes.

Minchin, Maureen, 1985 (2nd impression 1988), *Breastfeeding Matters*, Alma Publications, Wendouree, Vic., and George Allen & Unwin, North Sydney, NSW.

Jennifer comments:
An important breastfeeding text. Not a quick read but worth a look, especially if you are interested in breastfeeding from a political perspective.

Sears, B., 1999, *The Anti-Aging Zone*, HarperCollins, New York.

Kit comments:
Sears has refined his ideas considerably since The Zone *(1995) was published. Although frequently criticised as a high-protein diet, Sears' suggestions are exactly the same as the US and Australian RDAs. Recommendations for daily calorie intake are, however, explicitly low (1999), to achieve an anti-ageing effect, and hence are entirely unsuitable for pregnant and lactating women.*

Our website: <www.posture-and-flexibility.com.au>.

Kit comments:
*You will find many useful items here, including a Discussion Board where you can post your comments and questions. Readers will join in and comment, and might well be able to answer your questions better than we can. Companion volumes (*Overcome Neck & Back Pain, *and* Stretching & Flexibility*) and their videotapes and audiotapes can be previewed here. The site also has a list of endorsed P&F teachers, all around Australia, and a few overseas.*

CONTACT DETAILS

If you wish to contact us for more information on *Posture & Flexibility* in general, or for copies of our books, videotapes, and audiotapes, you can reach us as follows:

- Kit Laughlin: <kit.laughlin@anu.edu.au>
- Jennifer Cristaudo: <panoptis@mail.dynamite.com.au>
- Telephone contact for books, audiotapes and videotapes: 1800 800 590
- Our website: <www.posture-and-flexibility.com.au>

To accompany this book, *Stretching & Pregnancy*, we have an audiotape and a videotape.

The audiotape ('Take a Break') contains two recordings. Side A is the long version of the relaxation script (Kit's voice and effects), whereas Side B is the shorter version of the script (with Jennifer's voice).

The videotape features Jennifer teaching all the prenatal and postnatal exercises, shot in the *Posture & Flexibility* room at the Australian National University. You can order the tapes and additional copies of this book from the website directly, or from the 1800 800 590 number if you prefer.

INDEX OF MAJOR SUBJECTS

Photo Index

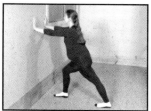

Ex. 1, p. 24

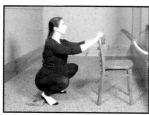

Ex. 2, p. 28

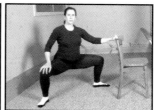

Ex. 3, p. 30

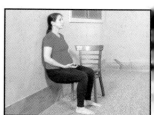

Ex. 4, p. 32

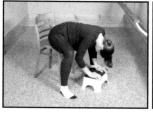

Ex. 5, p. 36

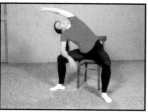

Ex. 6, p. 38

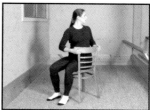

Ex. 7, p. 42

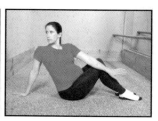

Ex. 8, p. 44

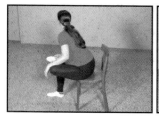

Ex. 9, p. 48

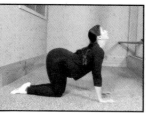

Ex. 10, p. 50

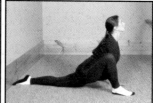

Ex. 11, p. 52

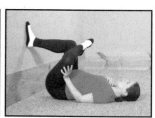

Ex. 12, p. 54

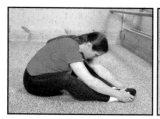

Ex. 13, p. 56

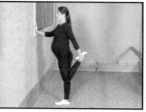

Ex. 14, p. 62

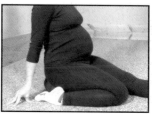

Ex. 15, p. 64

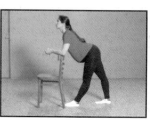

Ex. 16, p. 66

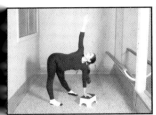

Ex. 17, p. 68

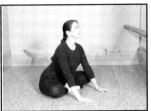

Ex. 18, p. 70

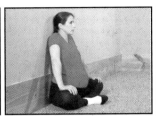

Ex. 19, p. 72

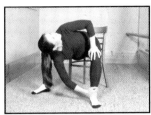

Ex. 20, p. 76

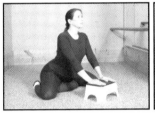

Ex. 21, p. 78

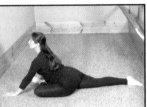

Ex. 22, p. 80

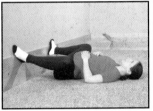

Ex. 23, p. 82

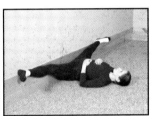

Ex. 24, p. 84

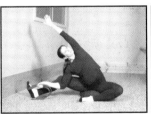

Ex. 25, p. 86

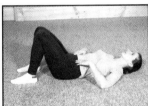

Ex. 26, p. 102

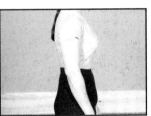

Ex. 27, p. 104

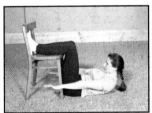

Ex. 28, p. 106

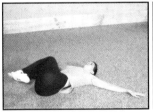

Ex. 29, p. 108

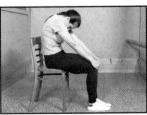

Ex. 30, p. 110

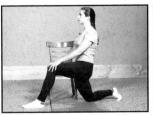

Ex. 31, p. 112

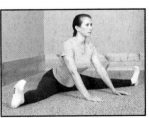

Ex. 32, p. 116